3
1/8/06

Skin Care in Wound Management: Assessment, prevention and treatment

Other titles available from Wounds UK include:

Honey: A modern wound management product
edited by Richard White, Rose Cooper and Peter Molan

Essential Wound Management: An introduction for undergraduates
edited by David Gray, Richard White and Pam Cooper

*Wound Healing: A systematic approach to advanced wound healing
and management* edited by David Gray, Richard White and Pam Cooper

A Pocket Guide to Clinical Decision-making in Wound Management
edited by David Gray and Sue Bale

Wounds UK — The Directory, 2006 edited by Richard White
and Clare Morris

Skin Care in Wound Management: Assessment, prevention and treatment

edited by

Richard White

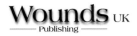
Wounds UK
Publishing

Wounds UK Publishing, Wounds UK Limited, Suite 3.1, 36 Upperkirkgate,
Aberdeen AB10 1BA

British Library Cataloguing-in-Publication Data
A catalogue record is available for this book

© Wounds UK Limited 2005
ISBN 0-9549193-3-5

Printed in the UK by Cromwell Press, Trowbridge, Wiltshire

CONTENTS

LIST OF CONTRIBUTORS

Sue Bale is Associate Director of Nursing, Gwent Healthcare NHS Trust, South Wales.

Martyn Butcher is Clinical Nurse Specialist, Tissue Viability, Derriford Hospital.

Michael Clark is Senior Research Fellow, Wound Healing Research Unit, Cardiff University.

Sylvie Hampton is Tissue Viability Consultant, Tissue Viability Consultancy Services Ltd (TVCS), Eastbourne.

Valerie Irving is Unit Manager, Neonatal Unit, Liverpool Women's Hospital.

Caroline McIntosh is Senior Lecturer in Podiatry, University of Huddersfield.

Clare Morris is Tissue Viability Advisor, North East Wales NHS Trust.

Veronica Newton is Senior Lecturer in Podiatry, University of Huddersfield.

Jackie Stephen-Haynes is Lecturer and Practitioner in Tissue Viability, Worcester University and Worcester Primary Care Trust.

Angela Vujnovich is Lead Nurse in Stoma Care, St Mark's and Northwich Park Hospital.

Richard White is a Clinical Research Consultant and Senior Research Fellow, Department of Tissue Viability, Aberdeen Royal Infirmary.

FOREWORD

The field of skin care and skin protection is central to the discipline of nursing. There are few nurses who do not have to address this issue in everyday practice, and for those working in the areas of dermatology, tissue viability, stoma care and continence, skin care is crucial to their practice.

This unique book fills an important need by addressing the clinical care relevant to many different aspects of nursing care. The text comprises previously unpublished material and tackles basic skin structure and function in an accessible fashion. This carefully selected collection of chapters, written by acknowledged experts in the field, addresses key issues in everyday skin care. The classification and management of superficial pressure ulcers is examined in detail, as is ulceration of the diabetic foot, the management of traumatic wounds, and neonatal skin care. All the chapters, including the one focusing on the link between incontinence damage and tissue breakdown and pressure ulceration, provide welcome reviews of the current evidence base and best practice. The chapter on stoma-related skin problems offers invaluable insights for non-specialist nurses, particularly in the community.

The importance of the nursing contribution to providing quality skin care and promoting skin health cannot be over-emphasised. This book will help to raise the profile of this often under-recognised area of care, which is so vital to patients' well-being.

Professor Dame Jill Macleod Clark DBE, PhD, RGN, FRGN
Head of School of Nursing and Midwifery
University of Southampton
October 2005

INTRODUCTION

There is common ground between dermatology, tissue viability, stoma care, podiatry and continence care. It is the protection of skin function in areas of risk, and, the management of skin already compromised by wound exudate, pressure, incontinence, or stoma leakage. We know that exudate can cause maceration which, in turn, leads to wound enlargement. Similarly, inadequate continence care leads to skin damage and can precipitate pressure ulceration. The early recognition of skin damage in the diabetic foot can, if managed appropriately, avoid deterioration into greater morbidity. The lesson is vigilance through observation and assessment: the remedy through evidence-based practice. The collection of chapters in this book is intended to address these areas by reference to current knowledge and best practice. Each chapter is written by an authority in the field, illustrated by clinical images and diagrams, and referenced comprehensively. The book is intended to guide and inform those practitioners who regularly encounter patients whose skin is at risk, or is already damaged, that constitute a large proportion of all patients throughout the age range.

Richard White
Whitstone
September 2005

CHAPTER 1

THE STRUCTURE AND FUNCTIONS OF THE SKIN

Martyn Butcher and Richard White

The healthy adult human skin is the largest organ of the body, providing about 10% of the body mass it covers an area of almost two square metres. Our skin has evolved to help us regulate heat and water loss, while acting as a barrier to the invasion by microorganisms and harmful chemicals. In this chapter we consider the detailed anatomy of each of the skin's layers, together with an overview of the major physiological and metabolic functions. It is intended to provide an insight into structure and function that will help the clinician understand the mechanisms of damage that might occur, and, the rationale for preventive and therapeutic interventions.

In gross terms, the skin comprises two major tissue layers, the cellular epidermis and the largely acellular dermis. Associated with these layers are a variety of appendages such as hair follicles, sweat glands, nerve endings and blood vessels.

The epidermis

The epidermis is the superficial cellular layer of the skin (*Figure 1.1*). Over most of the body surface it is very thin — about 0.1mm — but on specially adapted areas such as the palmar and plantar surfaces it can be 1mm–2mm thick. These areas are recognised as being 'extra protective', designed for walking and handling; this thickened tissue is the end product of epidermal cell differentiation. The epidermis has no direct blood supply, it receives all of its nutrients and oxygen by diffusion from the vascular network in the superficial (papillary) dermis. The epidermis comprises a number of cell layers (*Figure 1.2*), each being a stage in the differentiation process of the major epidermal cell — the keratinocyte. These cells make up about 95% of the epidermal cell population, the others being melanocytes, Langerhans cells and Merkel cells.

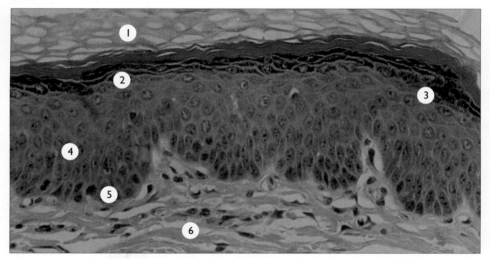

Figure 1.1: Histology of typical epidermis and superficial dermis
1. Stratum dysjunctum; 2. Stratum compactum (these two together form the stratum corneum); 3. Stratum granulosum (granular layer); 4. Stratum spinosum; 5. Stratum basale (basal layer); 6. Stratum (papillary) dermis

Epidermal cells

The keratinocyte is a typical epithelial cell, forming the lining of all internal and external body surfaces, eg. mucosal tissues. The epidermis is a stratified epithelium. Keratinocytes begin life from cell division at the basement membrane level, and, as they slowly migrate towards the skin surface, differentiate to become 'spinous' or 'prickle' cells, then 'granular' cells (both due to the microscopic appearance) and, finally, squames or stratum corneum cells. This process is accompanied by biochemical and morphological changes; each designed to modify the cell for its eventual role in physical protection and permeability barrier function. The newly formed basal keratinocyte is very much like any other epithelial cell in appearance, but as it migrates its appearance changes. The spinous cell is so-called because of the histological appearance of its numerous junctions (desmosomes) with neighbouring cells (*Figure 1.2*). These cell junctions affix the basal cells firmly to the basement membrane, and, in the layers up to the corneum, each cell to another. The end result is an epidermis that resists shear forces. The production of keratin protein and keratohyaline granules, known as 'keratinisation', within the cell, gives the stratum granulosum cell its characteristic appearance (Matoltsy, 1975). This may be regarded as the last 'living' cell layer in the epidermis as, hereafter, cells enter the stratum corneum where they are little more than flattened sacs of inert protein, devoid of the nucleus and other organelles associated with living cells. The end stage of the life of the keratinocyte is known as desquamation — this is the orderly loss of cells from the skin surface once their purpose has been served. To illustrate the importance of this process, abnormal desquamation often presents as a disease state, as is the case with psoriasis and ichthyosis.

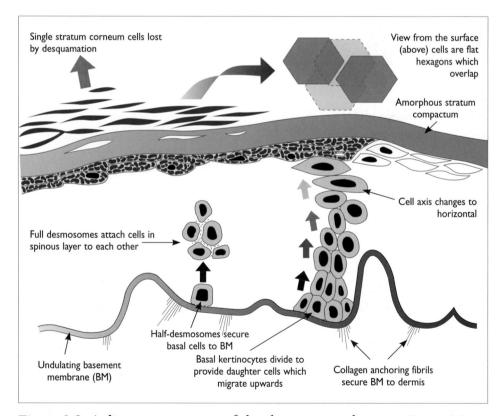

Figure 1.2: A diagrammatic view of the skin section, shown in *Figure 1.1* illustrating key features of epidermal biology

The melanocyte

The pigmentation of human and animal tissues not only provides cosmetic colouration to the skin, hair and eyes, but also gives significant protection to the body from ultra-violet (UV) radiation damage. Failure of this mechanism leads to photoaging and carcinogenesis (eg. melanoma). The melanocyte is the cell most closely associated with the pigmentary system. In the skin, this dendritic cell resides in the basal region of the epidermis, where it synthesises melanin pigment granules (as special organelles — melanosomes), and transfers them to neighbouring keratinocytes. These granules serve to disperse incident UV radiation, so protecting cell nuclei from damage (Hearing, 2005). The distribution of pigment also serves to give the skin and hair its colour (the hair bulb has a melanocyte population). Melanin synthesis is regulated by complex pathways of receptors and hormones (pituitary gland melanocyte-stimulating hormone or MSH; Slominski *et al*, 2004); it is triggered by exposure to UV radiation (sunlight) and hormones such as oestrogens and progestogens.

The Langerhans cell

The skin plays a key role in immune reactions to environmental antigens (see below for more details) and central to that is the Langerhans cell. This is a dendritic cell, derived from bone marrow leucocytes, which resides exclusively in the basal region of the epidermis. These cells are known as 'antigen presenting' cells, they transport antigens from the epidermis to draining lymph nodes (Romani *et al*, 2003). Antigens, such as microorganisms and foreign proteins, are presented to T helper lymphocytes. In so doing, Langerhans cells regulate processes such as the development of cytotoxic T lymphocytes, the production of antibodies by B lymphocytes, and, the activation of macrophages.

The Merkel cell

At the level of the stratum basale there is a population of 'neuroendocrine' cells which form a mechanoreceptor function — these are Merkel cells. Recent evidence shows that cutaneous tactile perception is due, in part, to the complex of Merkel cells and axon terminals of type 1 sensory nerve fibres (Ogawa, 1996; Johnson, 2001; Tachibana and Nawa, 2002). In addition, these cells have been claimed to regulate keratinocyte proliferation and differentiation, but this remains speculative at this time (Tachibana, 1995).

The basement membrane and dermo-epidermal junction

The interface between the epidermis and dermis is defined by a membrane, the basement membrane. This is made largely from collagens — the important connective tissue proteins (see below) — and provides a secure foundation for the basal keratinocytes, mechanical support for the epidermis, and a semi-permeable filter which regulates the passage of cells and nutrients from dermis to epidermis. The membrane itself is firmly attached to the dermis by means of more collagen-anchoring fibrils. The real value of this system of cell anchorage only becomes apparent in disease states, where its performance is compromised: thus, in the bullous diseases of pemphigus and pemphigoid, and in epidermolysis bullosa, defective basement membrane function leads to debilitating conditions.

Stratum corneum

The stratum corneum is often regarded as a homogeneous layer; it is however, two subtly different layers — the lower stratum compactum and the exterior stratum dysjunctum (Bowser and White, 1985). The compactum is the location of the water permeability barrier. Biochemical changes, particularly to lipids, occur as cells metamorphose from granular to compactum, providing the transient barrier property that is lost on conversion into the dysjunctum. The outermost dysjunctum is the interface with our environment; the cells here serve as a physical protective material. As they have no barrier capacity and are porous, they will readily absorb water — this is the effect we see as maceration. Palmar and plantar skin has a particularly thick stratum corneum, mostly dysjunctum, and is especially prone to maceration (White and Cutting, 2003).

The epidermal permeability barrier

The epidermal barrier property is one of 'controlled' water loss (from within), and of resistance to the ingress of microorganisms and noxious environmental chemicals. It is not a barrier in the sense that a sheet of plastic functions as a totally impervious barrier to gases and liquids. We lose water as vapour through the intact skin at a controlled rate; this is not sweat. It is known as transepidermal water loss or TEWL and acts in a fashion similar to the moisture vapour transmission (MVTR) from some semi-permeable wound dressings. The purpose is to maintain the superficial stratum corneum as a supple, pliable region. Dryness, whether clinical or sub-clinical, gives the skin a tight, rough feel. While the barrier can keep some chemicals out, its role in this capacity is not absolute. We know that some drugs, for example, corticosteroids and oestrogens, readily penetrate the skin in the context of 'transdermal drug delivery' (Hadgraft, 2004; Thomas and Finnin, 2004; Prausnitz *et al*, 2004).

Thus, the epidermis may be regarded as a tissue in dynamic equilibrium; with each cell division in the basal region, a dead cell is lost by desquamation from the surface — having contributed to the role as barrier and physical interface on the way (Madison, 2003).

The cutaneous immune system

At the interface with our environment, the skin is the tissue most often confronted with foreign antigens and pathogens (Bos, 1997; Misery, 1997). There are four typical immunological skin reactions: type I includes the immediate hypersensitivity reactions mediated by IgE and mast cells. These include anaphylaxis, angioedema, and wheal — flare (histamine release). Type II are the humoral-cytotoxic reactions mediated by complement, IgG and IgM. Type III reactions include vasculitis and type IV includes granulomatous reactions and delayed hypersensitivity. The dense network of epidermal Langerhans cells (see above) is associated with the skin-specific contact allergy known as delayed hypersensitivity (or type IV reaction). Practitioners in wound care will often see these reactions as allergies to adhesives, dressings and skin preparations common in patients with venous leg ulceration.

As this is such a complex area, the reader is recommended to consult specialist texts for further details, for example, Roitt IM and Delves JP, *Essential Immunology*, tenth edition, Blackwell Science Publishing, London.

The dermis

Underlying the basement membrane zone is the relatively acellular layer known as the dermis. This is a collection of cells and structures that fulfil many of the key functions of the skin, and is predominantly made up of the fibrous proteins, collagen and elastin. These form what is generally known as connective tissue. Suspended in these structures are supportive structures such as the vascular and neurological components. The dermis makes up 15%–20% of the total weight of the human body. It varies in thickness from approximately 5mm in areas such as the back and thighs, to as little as 1mm in the skin of the eyelids.

The dermis is regarded as two differing layers with subtle variations in composition, microscopic appearance, and function (*Figure 1.3*). The more superficial papillary dermis is found directly below the basement membrane. It is composed predominantly of a fine woven network of collagen fibres. These run around hair follicles and sebaceous glands, and around eccrine and apocrine glands, as well as between the rete ridges. This region is also rich in hyaluronic acid or hyaluronan. This is a carbohydrate polymer of glucuronic acid, which, in the dermis forms a viscous gel providing physical cushioning visco-elastic support (Balasz, 2004).

The reticular dermis forms the base of the dermal layer and is mainly made up of thicker bundles of collagen fibres.

During life, collagen is continually being broken down and replaced.

It is synthesised by cells known as dermal fibroblasts. These cells secrete tropocollagen which, after further extracellular processing, is converted to mature collagen. Normal adult human skin is made up of approximately 85% type I collagen and 15% type III collagen (Gay and Miller, 1978). In fetal life, type III collagen is far more common. These materials provide the skin with its tensile strength.

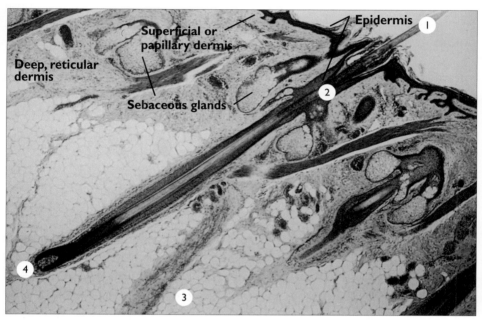

Figure 1.3: This transverse section of human skin shows an area rich in hair shafts and sebaceous glands. Note the scale of the hair, this provides a reference for the thickness of the epidermis. The high density of sebaceous glands is typical of facial or scalp tissues and will result in an oily/greasy skin. Note that the hair follicle is an invagination of the epidermis
1. Hair shaft emerges from the skin surface; 2. Sebaceous glands discharge sebum into the hair follicle; 3. Fat cells in sub-cutis; 4. The hair bulb

Elastin fibres are found throughout the dermis. These are also manufactured by the fibroblasts, but their main role is to provide the elastic recoil of the skin. This permits tissues to return to their relative positions after lateral stress, preventing the skin from becoming 'baggy'. Elastic fibres are thicker and more common in the lower levels of the dermis, however, their numbers do not remain constant throughout life. Elastic fibres degenerate with age and exposure to ultra-violet radiation.

This results in the classic sagging and stretching of the skin that we experience in old age.

The gaps between collagen bundles, collagen fibres and elastic fibres, are filled with a substance referred to as 'ground substance'. This acts as an amorphous filling agent.

Hair follicle

Hair follicles are first seen during the third month of fetal development. The hair follicle is made up of three areas. The lower section extends from the base of the follicle to the insertion of the erector pili muscle; the middle portion extends from the muscle to the entrance of the sebaceous gland; and the final portion extends from the sebaceous gland to the surface of the skin. The structure of the follicle changes with the growth cycle of the hair. In normal hair development the active growth phase lasts at least three years, with the regressive phase lasting about three weeks and the resting period lasting approximately three months. At any one time, about 84% of hair follicles are in the active growth phase (Thiers and Galbraith, 1986).

The hair follicle is lined with epidermal cells and is a downward extension, or invagination, of the epidermis. Although the bulk of this structure is found in the dermis, it should be considered an epidermal component. In the lower portion of the follicle, cells form the hair matrix from which the hair itself develops. There are a number of melanocytes found in this area. These are responsible for the production of hair colour. As cells migrate upwards they differentiate and keratinise, the outer layers in each hair hardening first.

Sebaceous glands

Sebaceous glands are found in skin throughout the body except on the palms of the hand and soles of the feet. In most areas they are associated with hair follicles, though in a few areas, notably the areolae, nipples, labia and inner prepuce they may be found as free structures. Their role is to produce the lipid-rich secretion sebum. These glands are present at birth but vary in size and action throughout life as a result of hormone stimulation. At birth, sebaceous glands are well-developed and active. This is probably the result of maternal hormone stimulation. Within months, the glands atrophy until puberty when, under the influence of androgens, glands increase in size and sebum production. At this time they are particularly active in facial skin and in the skin of the nose.

Sweat glands: eccrine and apocrine

Eccrine glands primarily serve in the regulation of body temperature through the production of sweat (Sato *et al*, 1995). The gland is formed of a tight coil which lies in the lower third of the dermis, but which may extend down as far as the dermal-subcutaneous fat level. A duct leads from the coil through to a downward projection of the rete ridges and then finally out onto the surface of the epidermis. The upper portions of this track are lined with epidermal cells, lower structures contain a secretory cell lining. On average, there are three million sweat glands in the human skin. These are capable of producing a maximum of 1.8 litres of sweat per hour. This consists of water, salts (predominantly sodium and potassium), as well as numerous proteolytic enzymes, indicating that sweat may possess pro-inflammatory or protective functions, as well as being involved in heat regulation.

Apocrine glands are found in distinct areas of the human skin. They are the equivalent of scent glands in humans and are only found in the axillae, in the anogenital region, and as modified glands in the external ear canal, in the eyelid and in the breast. Although present at birth, they only begin their secretory action after puberty.

Blood vessels

The blood vessels of the dermis are divided into two planes. The superficial vascular plexus is made up of interconnecting arterioles and venules which lie close to the epidermal border and wrap around the structures of the dermis such as hair follicles. These supply oxygen and nutrients to these rapidly metabolising cells. There is a second network known as the deep vascular plexus. This is found deeper in the dermis at its border to the subcutaneous fat layer. It is made up of more substantial vessels. Vertical vessels connect these two plexus.

The glomus cells are specialised vascular structures that are found in the reticular dermis, mainly in the pads of the fingers and toes, but also in the volar aspect of the hands and feet and in the central facial region. They represent areas of arteriovenous shunting that do not have a capillary network between the arterioles and venules, and are concerned with temperature regulation. When opened, these areas permit the rapid transfer of blood which aids in radiant heat loss.

Mast cells

These cells are part of the immune system. Mast cells are found around blood vessels, nerves and appendages in the dermis, predominantly in the region of the dermal vascular plexus (Eady, 1976). They contain a number of granules. These are extruded from the cell after cross-linking with IgE on the cell surface. Degranulation occurs within minutes of exposure to the stimulant, releasing a number of molecules, including histamine. In the skin, this produces relaxation of smooth muscle causing vasodilation. Histamine also increases capillary permeability attracting more leukocytes to the affected area. In time, the mast cells produce inflammatory mediators — prostaglandins and leukotrienes, as well as a variety of cytokines that promote the inflammatory process. In addition, mast cells secrete tumour necrosis factor-α (TNF-α), which acts as a chemo-attractant to neutrophils.

Neural network

It is believed that around one million afferent nerve fibres innervate the skin (Sinclair, 1981). The skin is supplied with both sensory and autonomic nerves. The autonomic nerves derive from the sympathetic nervous system and supply the blood vessels, erector pili muscles, eccrine and apocrine glands. Sebaceous glands show an absence of autonomic pathways, relying on endocrine stimulation to activate their function.

Sensory nerves enter the skin at the sub-dermal fatty tissue, each dividing into smaller bundles that fan out in a horizontal plane to form a branching network. These fibres ascend to the superficial dermal layers. Most end in the dermis, however, a number penetrate into the basement membrane. There are a number of different types of sensory receptors in the skin, each one developed to react to one form of external stimuli. The sensations of touch, pressure, heat and cold, and pain are mediated by the dendritic endings of different sensory neurons.

The sensation of heat and cold are mediated by simple neurons. The receptors for cold are located in the dermis just below the epidermal junction. They are stimulated by cooling and inhibited by warming. Receptors for heat are located deeper in the dermis and are fewer in number. Exposure to very high temperatures also produces the sensation of pain. This occurs as a result of the activation of a particular protein — a capsaicin receptor. High temperatures or exposure to capsaicin, the chemical in chilli peppers which causes the 'burn', results in ion channels being opened. This permits the diffusion of Ca^{2+} and Na^+ ions into the neuron producing depolarisation. This ultimately stimulates the central nervous system permitting the perception of heat and pain.

Pain is also perceived through action of specialist pain receptors. These naked receptors transmit electrical activity through the axon to the spinal cord where they synapse, and the stimuli is transmitted to the higher centres of the brain. Sharp pain sensations are transmitted through myelinated axons, capable of transmitting impulses rapidly; whereas dull pain and ache is transmitted via slower non-myelinated axons. There is evidence that adenosine triphosphate released from damaged cells, along with a local fall in pH (for instance, following inflammation and infection), also stimulate these receptors — leading to pain.

Touch sensations are mediated through simple nerve endings surrounding hair follicles, and specialist nerve endings called Merkel's discs and Ruffini endings. Touch and pressure are also mediated by dendrites encapsulated within various structures, including Meissner's corpuscles and pacinian corpuscles. These structures are found in the dermis throughout the individual, but are most heavily concentrated in the hands and feet, particularly in the finger tips.

Muscle cells

The dermis contains a number of muscle fibres. Smooth involuntary muscle makes up the erector pili apparatus which is responsible for elevating body hair, producing goose-bumps, but is also found in the nipple. Striated muscle is found in the neck (platysma) and in the face where it controls fine facial movement and facial expression.

Lymphatic system

In normal conditions the skin has a rich lymphatic system. This is responsible for the transportation of particulate and liquid material, such as protein from the extravascular compartment of the dermis. Broad lumen vessels with single cell thick walls transport fluid away from the skin and to the lymph nodes, maintaining homeostasis in the tissues.

Skin functions

Temperature regulation

In evolutionary terms, the development of warm-blooded animals had a significant impact on the animal world and the evolution of the mammals. Through the maintenance of a relatively constant core temperature it was possible to maintain rapid cell metabolism regardless of climatic conditions. This, however, does have a major problem; the need to preserve heat and dissipate excess heat energy as the need arose.

As already indicated, the neural network of the skin provides man with an accurate measure of ambient temperature through the activation of heat and cold receptors in the dermis. Signals are passed via the nerve pathways to the hypothalamus, which can initiate the inhibition of sweating or the initiation of shivering. However, ambient stimuli have relatively little influence on core body temperature other than getting us to reach for that extra layer of clothing.

What does have a significant effect is the major role the skin plays in direct thermoregulation. Excess heat can be lost through the skin by conduction, convection, radiation and evaporation. Sweating, a function of the eccrine glands, permits the dissipation of excess heat energy by evaporation; while the dilation and constriction of the rich blood vessels in the dermal plexus enables heat energy to be modified in the underlying structures. Damage to this skin function, through burns or inflammatory conditions such as severe eczema and Steven-Johnson syndrome, can lead to catastrophic collapse and is often referred to as skin failure (Irvine, 1991).

Vitamin D synthesis

The production of 1,25-dihydroxyvitamin D_3 begins in the skin where vitamin D_3 is produced from its precursor molecule under the influence of sunlight. Vitamin D_3 is an essential component in calcium regulation in the body and so affects bone deposition and serum calcium levels. It has also been postulated that it acts as an autocrine regulator of the epidermis. This idea is supported by the action of UV light and vitamin D analogues on the skin in patients suffering from psoriasis, where it inhibits cell proliferation and promotes differentiation of keratinocytes, (Fox, 2002).

Protection against UV radiation

As well as visible light, the sun produces a range of radiation that is invisible to the naked eye, but which has an effect on the function of the skin. Ultra-violet (UV) light is made up of two main wave bands. The shorter wavelength UVB rays are able to penetrate the epidermis and cause sunburn and, in the long term, skin cancer. Longer wavelength UVA rays are believed to be the major cause of skin changes associated with ageing.

The skin has two methods of protection against UV radiation; a pigmentation barrier formed by melanin, and a protein barrier found in the stratum corneum. Both act by minimising the absorption of harmful radiation by cellular DNA, therefore minimising the genetic mutation potential.

Communication

In many ways the skin can be viewed as a 'window to the soul'. Owing to the influence that systemic disease can have on the appearance of the skin, whether through colour, texture, temperature or function, clinicians can use it as an indicator of inner body functions and well-being of the individual — as a way of assessing general health and diagnosing disease. As such, clinicians need to be able to recognise normal and abnormal cutaneous phenomena that present themselves: they need to learn to read the signs.

Outside the purely medical context, while it may appear obvious, the skin is the one structure we see when we communicate with other humans. In particular, facial movement and expression is used by humans as a method of communicating mood, emotion, and as a primary method of identification. The ability to influence sensation through touch is used as a primary method of expressing bonding, love, aggression, concern and friendship. Changes in the function or appearance of the skin can have profound effects on how we perceive those around us and ourselves. Features such as skin blemishes, disease scars and other stigmata can be influential on interpersonal relationships and issues of self-image.

References

Balasz EA (2004) The viscoelastic properties of hyaluronan and its therapeutic use. In: Garg H, Hales C, eds. _Chemistry and Biology of Hyaluronan_. Elsevier publications, London: chap 20

Bos JD (1997) The skin as an organ of immunity. _Clin Exp Immunol_ **107**: suppl 1: 3–5

Bowser PA, White RJ (1985) Isolation, barrier properties and lipid analysis of stratum compactum, a discrete region of stratum corneum. _Br J Dermatol_ **112**: 1–14

Eady RAJ (1976) The mast cells: distribution and morphology. _Clin Exp Dermatol_ **1**: 313–21

Fox SI (2002) Regulation of metabolism. 7th edn. _Human Physiology_. McGraw Hill, London: 607

Gay S, Miller S (1978) _Collagen in the Physiology and Pathology of Connective Tissue_. Gustav Fischer Verlag, Stuttgart

Hadgraft J (2004) Skin deep. *Eur J Pharm Biopharm* **58**(2): 291–9

Hearing VJ (2005) Biogenesis of pigment granules: a sensitive way to regulate melanocyte function. *J Dermatol Sci* **37**(1): 3–14

Irvine C (1991) 'Skin Failure' — a real entity: discussion paper. *J Roy Soc Med* **84**: 412–3

Johnson KO (2001) The roles and functions of cutaneous mechanoreceptors. *Curr Opin Neurobiol* **114**: 455–61

Madison KC (2003) Barrier function of the skin: 'la raison d'etre' of the epidermis. *J Invest Dermatol* **121**(2): 231–42

Matoltsy AG (1975) Desmosomes, filaments, and keratohyaline granules: their role in the stabilisation and keratinization of the epidermis. *J Invest Dermatol* **65**(1): 127–42

Misery L (1997) Skin, immunity and the nervous system. *Br J Dermatol* **137**(6): 843–50

Ogawa H (1996) The Merkel cell as a possible mechanoreceptor cell. *Prog Neurobiol* **49**(4): 317–34

Prausnitz MR, Mitragotri S, Langer R (2004) Current status and future potential of transdermal drug delivery. *Nat Rev Drug Discov* **3**(2): 115–24

Romani N, Holzmann S, Tripp CH *et al* (2003) Langerhans cells — dendritic cells of the epidermis. *APMIS* **111**(7/8): 725–40

Sato K (1977) The physiology, pharmacology, and biochemistry of the eccrine sweat gland. *Rev Physiol Biochem Pharmacol* **79**: 51–131

Sinclair DC (1981) *Mechanisms of Cutaneous Sensation.* 2nd edn. Oxford University Press, Oxford

Slominski A, Tobin DJ *et al* (2004) Melanin pigmentation in mammalian skin and its hormonal regulation. *Physiol Rev* **84**(4): 1155–228

Tachibana T (1995) The Merkel cell: recent findings and unresolved problems. *Arch Histol Cytol* **58**(4): 379–96

Tachibana T, Nawa T (2002) Recent progress in studies on Merkel cell biology. *Anat Sci Int* **77**(1): 26–33

Thiers BH, Galbraith GMP (1986) Alopaecia areata. In: Thiers BH, Dobson RL, eds. *Pathogenesis of Skin Diseases.* Churchill Livingstone, New York: 57

Thomas BJ, Finnin BC (2004) The transdermal revolution. *Drug Discov Today* **15**(9): 697–703

White RJ, Cutting KF (2003) Interventions to avoid maceration of the skin and wound bed. *Br J Nurs* **12**(20): 1186–1201

Windoffer R, Borchert-Stuhltrager M, Leube RF (2002) Desmosomes. *J Cell Sci* **115**(8): 1717–32

CHAPTER 2

SUPERFICIAL PRESSURE ULCERS

Michael Clark and Jackie Stephen-Haynes

Part I: The nature of the problem

Pressure ulcers continue to puzzle, tantalise and often frustrate. Despite numerous initiatives and the widespread adoption of pressure-redistributing devices, there is no firm evidence that these strategies and tactics (with their associated cost) have reduced the number of people who experience pressure ulcers in healthcare settings (Clark and Orchard, 2004). This is not to say that the interventions used are ineffective, but rather that fundamental questions remain unaddressed — for example, when is a pressure ulcer not a pressure ulcer? Such questions relate to the clinical significance of the early stages of pressure ulcers and this chapter will explore the classification and epidemiology of superficial pressure ulcers.

Background

Pressure ulcers, venous leg ulcers and diabetic foot ulcers are usually considered to be the three main groups of chronic wounds. Such a statement contains hidden assumptions regarding both the aetiology and clinical presentation of each type of chronic wound. For example, if pressure ulcers are, indeed, a single wound type, then each 'pressure ulcer' should share a common aetiology and manifest with relatively similar appearance. At least with regard to their clinical presentation, this assumption does not hold true with pressure ulcers ranging from localised areas of discoloured skin, through to large cavity wounds involving all tissues, including bone. Less is known regarding the mechanisms through which pressure ulcers arise, but there is a general awareness that some pressure ulcers may arise due to direct skin and soft tissue compression, while others may be the consequence of forces acting parallel to the skin surface (shear forces). So, both in terms of their aetiology and clinical presentation, pressure ulcers do not form a homogeneous wound type. Given this, discussion of pressure ulceration may be best advanced through appropriate classification of the wide range of manifestations of wounds caused by excessive or prolonged mechanical loading of the skin and soft tissues.

Aware of the need to classify pressure ulcers but confused as to how to describe these wounds?

This awareness that there is a need for pressure ulcer classification is relatively recent; in 1975 the first pressure ulcer conference to be held in the United Kingdom made no mention of any pressure ulcer classification schemes (Kenedi *et al*, 1976). In the same year, Shea (1975) published a seminal report separating pressure ulcers into five types (*Table 2.1*). Following Shea's initial classification, several authors attempted to modify pressure ulcer classification primarily to improve the ability to discriminate between undamaged skin and the first stages of pressure damage (*Table 2.2*). *Table 2.2* highlights the confusion within pressure ulcer classification schemes based solely upon their appearance. Some classification schemes include potential necrotic areas as the earliest stage of pressure ulcer (eg. David *et al*, 1983), while, in others, there are discrepancies between the limit of tissue damage that marks a grade II pressure ulcer (in some, eg. Versluysen [1986] only the epidermis is damaged, while in other schemes, eg. Yarkony *et al* [1990] the damage may also extend into the dermis).

In 1992, Clark and Cullum were the first to describe grade I and II pressure ulcers as being 'superficial', with other grades being described as being 'severe' pressure ulcers. This discrimination between superficial and severe marks both the general appearance of the wounds, the tissue layers involved in the injury, and also reflects Shea's (1975) observation that early stages of pressure damage were reversible, while more severe forms required aggressive intervention to repair the tissue damage.

Table 2.1: Pressure ulcer classification as described by Shea (1975). The descriptions of each grade are taken directly from Shea (1975)

Pressure ulcer grade	Description of tissue damage relevant to each grade
I	'Irregular, ill-defined area of soft tissue swelling and induration with associated heat and erythema overlying a bony prominence'. Can also present as a 'moist superficial irregular ulceration limited to the epidermis exposing the underlying dermis and resembling an abrasion'.
II	'Shallow full-thickness skin ulcer whose edges are more distinct with early fibrosis and pigmentation changes blending into a broad indistinct area of heat, erythema and induration'. Grades I and II were considered by Shea to be reversible wounds.
III	'Irregular full-thickness skin defect extending into the subcutaneous fat exposing a draining, foul-smelling, infected, necrotic base which has undermined the skin for a variable distance.'
IV	Appearance 'resembles that of a Grade III except that bone can be identified in the base of the ulceration which is more extensively undermined with profuse drainage and necrosis.'
Closed pressure ulcer	'Unremarkable in its presentation with a small benign-appearing ulcer measuring a few millimeters in diameter... with minimal drainage' these wounds hide necrosis in the subcutaneous fat.

Table 2.2: Definitions of grade I and II pressure ulcers from selected publications issued between 1976 and 1992

Author(s)	Definition of grade I	Definition of grade II
Jordan and Clark (1977)	Skin discoloration	Superficial pressure ulcer
David et al (1983)	Where the skin is likely to break down (red, black and blistered areas). Healed areas still covered by a scab	Superficial break in the skin
Versluysen (1986)	Persistent discolouration at same site for at least 48 hours, also blister	Epidermal loss only
NPUAP (1989)	Non-blanchable erythema of intact skin	Partial-thickness skin loss involving epidermis and/or dermis
Yarkony et al (1990)	Red area; present longer than 30 minutes, but less than 24 hours; present longer than 24 hours	Epidermis and/or dermis ulcerated with no subcutaneous fat observed
Clark and Cullum (1992)	Non-blanchable erythema	Superficial break in the skin

Recent trends and new initiatives in the classification of superficial pressure ulcers

From the early 1990s, the classification of early or superficial pressure ulcers appeared to focus upon grade I marking changes in intact skin, whereas grade II denoted a breach of the epidermis but where the damage did not extend into the subcutaneous fat (National Pressure Ulcer Advisory Panel [NPUAP], 1989; European Pressure Ulcer Advisory Panel [EPUAP], 1999). For example, part of the EPUAP definition of a grade I pressure ulcer is 'non-blanchable erythema of intact skin'. During the 1990s, visually-based pressure ulcer classifications were questioned about their relevance when assessing darkly-pigmented skin (for example, Lyder, 1996). These observations led to a redefinition of grade I pressure ulcers to include indicators other than skin colour changes. For example, the United States NPUAP amended its definition of a grade I pressure ulcer in 1997 to read:

> *A stage I pressure ulcer is an observable pressure-related alteration of intact skin whose indicators as compared to the adjacent or opposite area on the body may include changes in one or more of the following: skin temperature (warmth or coolness), tissue consistency (firm or boggy feel), and/or sensation (pain, itching).*

The ulcer appears as a defined area of persistent redness in lightly pigmented skin, whereas in darker skin tones, the ulcer may appear with persistent red, blue, or purple hues. In a similar revision, the EPUAP added other characteristics of early pressure ulcers to their visually-based definition of a grade I pressure ulcer:

> *Discolouration of the skin, warmth, oedema, induration or hardness may also be used as indicators (beyond non-blanchable erythema), particularly on individuals with darker skin.*

The cynical may suggest that these recent changes to the definitions of grade I pressure ulcers help to complete the circle by bringing the grade I pressure ulcer definition largely back to the proposal of Shea (1975, *Table 2.1*).

Recently, both the NPUAP and EPUAP have again explored the definitions of early stage pressure ulcers; the EPUAP focused upon the discrimination between pressure-induced grade II ulcers and similar wounds resulting from the abrasion of moist skin (Defloor *et al*, 2005).

The potential role of moisture in creating the wounds we often refer to as superficial pressure ulcers is not a new observation. Clark (1996) reported upon the fate of ninety elderly hospital patients of whom eleven developed pressure ulcers during their stay in hospital (six developed grade I or II sacral pressure ulcers). Of the ninety subjects, forty-six remained free from pressure ulcers while in hospital. A series of biomechanical and physiological measurements were recorded at the sacrum of the ninety subjects, and these measurements were used to discriminate between the ulcer-free group and those who developed superficial sacral wounds. All measurements were made before any visible signs of pressure damage at the sacrum. Measurement of contact pressure between the sacrum and the bed surface did not help to discriminate between those who developed superficial sacral pressure ulcers, and those who remained free of these wounds, suggesting that mechanical loading may not have been the primary cause of these wounds. However, the skin of those who subsequently developed superficial sacral pressure ulcers was moister than that of those who remained free from pressure ulcers, indicating that moisture may be a significant causal factor when considering superficial pressure ulcers. The recent position paper from the EPUAP (Defloor _et al_, 2005) extends this observation by providing assistance to clinicians to discriminate pressure- and moisture-induced grade II wounds based upon their location and appearance.

The NPUAP, meanwhile, have recently returned to the classification of grade I pressure ulcers looking at the inclusion of wounds similar to Shea's closed pressure ulcers within the grade I classification (Clark, 2005). These recent attempts to refine further the definitions of superficial pressure ulcers clearly illustrate that the identification of superficial pressure ulcers remains challenging, and that the confusion evident within the first classification schemes remains largely unresolved.

Epidemiology of superficial pressure ulcers

In 2001, the EPUAP conducted a pilot pressure ulcer prevalence survey across twenty-six hospitals located in five countries (Belgium, Italy, Portugal, Sweden and the United Kingdom) (Clark _et al_, 2004). Of the 5947 surveyed patients, 1078 (18.1%) had pressure ulcers at the time of the survey. Of these, 454 (42.1%) and 282 (26.1%) had grade I or II pressure ulcers respectively. That the majority of encountered pressure ulcers are superficial has been reported by several authors across a wide range of countries (for example, Lahmann *et al*, 2005 [Germany], Conzut *et al*, 2002 [Italy], Barczak *et al*, 1997 [USA], Lepisto *et al*, 2001 [Finland], among many others). While these surveys consistently indicate the high numbers of people with superficial pressure ulcers in hospital, there remains debate regarding whether all superficial pressure ulcers should be included in prevalence or incidence studies. This debate dates back to the first prevalence surveys conducted in the United Kingdom (Barbenel *et al*, 1977), and centres upon the ability of health professionals to correctly identify early stages of pressure ulcer — the belief being that grade I pressure ulcers are frequently under-reported. Jordan and Clark (1977) reported that inter-observer reliability when identifying grade I and II pressure ulcers was calculated during the first UK large-scale pressure ulcer prevalence survey (Barbenel *et al*, 1977). In this study, 5% of the wards surveyed were assessed by a team of seven nurses who had not participated in the prevalence survey. These wards had reported 171 pressure ulcers during the survey, while the independent team found 208 wounds, an overall reporting accuracy of 82.2%. When the accuracy of reporting was considered by grade of pressure ulcer, there were 122 and 142 reported and observed grade I pressure ulcers respectively (85.9% reporting accuracy). The accuracy of reporting pressure ulcers fell when wounds that involved a breach in the skin were considered (grades II and above), with forty-nine reported and sixty-six observed (74.2% accuracy of reporting). Other large-scale surveys found very different reporting accuracies by grade of pressure ulcer. David *et al* (1983) visited sixty wards marking 8% of their entire survey population; on these wards, 47/888 patients had been reported to have pressure ulcers but 64 pressure ulcer patients were observed; a 73% reporting accuracy. When this was explored by grade of pressure ulcer, only 30% of existing grade I pressure ulcers were reported; while the accuracy of reporting wounds where the skin was broken exceeded 80%. It would appear that grade I pressure ulcers may be under-reported in some surveys but not in all. However, where under-reporting exists, then its magnitude (as shown in David *et al*, 1983) may be such as to markedly under-estimate the true scale of the problem of pressure ulcers. Defloor *et al* (2005) recommended that data upon all grades of pressure ulcer be collected during prevalence and incidence surveys, but that only data upon grades II through to IV should be used to calculate prevalence proportions and incidence rates. The value of collecting data upon grade I pressure ulcers rests upon their role as 'warning signs' that preventive action should be initiated. So, in this recent position paper, the EPUAP appears to answer the question posed in the introduction to this section — a pressure ulcer is not a pressure ulcer when it presents as an area of unbroken but discoloured skin. This is probably not the end of the debate regarding the clinical relevance of superficial pressure ulcers, but merely represents another stage on our exploration of the phenomenon of skin and soft tissue pressure-induced damage.

References

Barbenel JC, Jordan MM, Nicol SM, Clark MO (1977) Incidence of pressure sores in the Greater Glasgow Health Board area. *Lancet* **2**(8037): 548–50

Barczak CA, Barnett RI, Childs EJ, Bosley LM (1997) Fourth national pressure ulcer prevalence survey. *Adv Wound Care* **10**(4): 18–26

Clark M, Orchard H (2004) Do we take pressure ulcers seriously enough? *J Tissue Viability* **14**(1): 2

Clark M (1996) The aetiology of superficial sacral pressure sores. In: Leaper DL, Cherry GW, Dealey C, eds. Proceedings of the 6th European Conference on Advances in Wound Management, Amsterdam. Macmillan Press: 167–9

Clark M (2005) What drives pressure ulcer classification — scientific knowledge or fear of litigation? *J Tissue Viability* **15**(2): 2,4

Clark M, Cullum N (1992) Matching patient need for pressure sore prevention with the supply of pressure-redistributing mattresses. *J Adv Nurs* **17**: 310–16

Clark M, Bours G, Defloor T (2004) A pilot study of the prevalence of pressure ulcers in European Hospitals. In: Clark M, ed. *Pressure Ulcers: Recent advances in tissue viability*. Quay Books, MA Healthcare Ltd, London

Conzut L, Bin A, Toneatto M, Quattrin R (2002) The surveillance system of decubital lesions of the University Polyclinic in Udine: results of an incidence study. *Assist Inferm Ric* **21**(1): 17–21

David JA, Chapman RG, Chapman EJ, Lockett B (1983) An investigation of the current methods used in nursing for the care of patients with established pressure sores. Final report to the Department of Health. Northwick Park, Nursing Practice Research Unit

Defloor T, Clark M, Witherow A, Colin D, Lindholm C, Schoonhoven L, Moore Z (2005) EPUAP statement on prevalence and incidence monitoring of pressure ulcer occurrence. *J Tissue Viability* **15**(3): 20–7

European Pressure Ulcer Advisory Panel (1999) Guidelines on treatment of pressure ulcers. *EPUAP Review* **1**(2): 136–69

Jordan MM, Clark MO (1977) Report on the incidence of pressure sores in the patient community of the Greater Glasgow Health Board Area on 21st January, 1976. University of Strathclyde, Glasgow

Kenedi RM, Cowden JM, Scales JT, eds (1976) *Bedsore Biomechanics.*
    Macmillan Press, London
Lahmann NA, Halfens RJ, Dassen T (2005) Prevalence of pressure ulcers in
    Germany. *J Clin Nurs* **14**(2): 165–72
Lepisto M, Eriksson E, Hietanen H, Asko-Seljavaara S (2001) Patients with
    pressure ulcers in Finnish hospitals. *Int J Nurs Pract* **7**(4): 280–7
Lyder CH (1996) Examining the inclusion of ethnic minorities in pressure
    ulcer prediction studies. *J Wound Ostomy Continence Nurs* **23**(5): 257–60
National Pressure Ulcer Advisory Panel (1989) Pressure ulcers: incidence,
    economics, risk assessment. Consensus development conference
    statement. *Decubitus* **2**(2): 24–8
Shea JD (1975) Pressure sores. Classification and management. *J Clin Orthop
    Related Res* **112**: 89–100
Versluysen M (1986) *Pathogenesis of pressure sores in elderly patients with hip
    fractures.* City and Hackney Health Authority, London
Yarkony GM, Kirk PM, Carlson C, Roth EJ, Lovell L, Heinemann A *et al*
    (1990) Classification of pressure ulcers. *Arch Dermatol* **126**(9): 1218–9

Part II: Practical issues

This part explores the important issues of understanding the development, assessment, and management issues surrounding superficial pressure ulcers. The recently published National Guidelines (National Institute for Clinical Excellence [NICE], 2005), clearly states that the presence of superficial pressure damage, grades I and II, is the greatest risk for higher grade pressure ulcer development. This issue is also given high priority in the Scottish Best Practice Statements (Nursing and Midwifery Practice Development Unit [NMPDU], 2002, 2005).

Superficial pressure ulcer development

The physiological development of pressure ulcers is subject to debate (NPUAP, 1989; EPUAP, 1999; Morison, 2001; Russell, 2003; Satsue, 2005). The tissue involved in pressure ulcer development is skin, subcutaneous fat, deep fascia, muscle and bone (Morison, 2001).

Pressure damage occurs over a boney prominence where body weight is concentrated; it can occur under a cast, splint, or anything that is compressed against the skin.

Normally, vascular and lymph vessels carry nutrients and oxygen to support cell metabolism, epidermal mitosis, facilitating temperature regulation and removal of waste products. Pressure ulcers develop as a result of two processes:

- the occlusion of blood vessels by external pressure and
- damage to the micro-circulation due to shearing and disruptive forces.

Factors influencing pressure ulcer development

Both intrinsic and extrinsic factors can lead to pressure ulcer development. Intrinsic factors include pressure, shear, friction, moisture, and the tolerance of the skin.

Intrinsic factors

❖ **Pressure**

It is often quoted that an external pressure greater than 32mmHg, considered the mean capillary pressure, will lead to capillary closure and damage. When capillary occlusion occurs, it may initially be seen as a reddened or shiny area, blister or epidermal breakdown. The pressure that leads to vascular occlusion, assumed to be 32mmHg, is increasingly subject to debate (Bridel, 1993).

❖ **Shear**

Shear forces are uniaxial forces which can cause tissue deformation leading to tissue damage and small blood vessel disruption. These forces are exerted when, for example, patients slide down, or are dragged up a bed or chair (Collins, 2002). When a high level of shear is present, the amount of external pressure leading to vascular occlusion is reduced by half (Bennett and Lee, 1985).

* **Friction**

Friction occurs when two surfaces move across one another. Poor lifting and handling techniques increase the risk of friction damage to the skin, potentially removing the top layers.

* **Moisture**

The causes of moist skin include incontinence, sweating, or wound exudate. Clark (1996) observed that the number of patients who developed superficial pressure ulcers was largely attributed to skin moisture, rather than mechanical loading to the skin. Clever *et al* (2002) stated that pressure damage is twenty-two times more likely when the patient is incontinent and, therefore, assessment of the cause of incontinence is essential with referral to a continence nurse if necessary. The natural changes that occur in the skin with age increase the risk of pressure damage. Normally, the skin acts as a barrier by repelling water, with the slightly acidic pH protecting from microorganisms and pathogenic bacteria that live on the skin. It is well-recognised that incontinence is a key causative factor in pressure ulcer development. This is explored in *Chapter 5*.

Excoriation can occur when the tissue is infiltrated and an inflammatory response is initiated. This can be extremely painful for the patient and can lead to pressure damage. Good preventative care and the use of a barrier film can protect the skin (Lewis-Byers *et al*, 2002). Diarrhoea can be particularly corrosive to the skin; such corrosion leads to irritation and excoriation. This can feel sore and uncomfortable for the patient, leading to skin breakdown and superficial pressure ulcer development. A barrier film is effective in minimising and preventing damage where an outbreak does occur (Butcher, 2002; Lewis-Byers *et al*, 2002; Schuren *et al*, 2005). Moisture and incontinence are significant causal factors when considering many superficial pressure ulcers.

* **Previous pressure ulceration**

Any patient with a history of pressure ulceration is at risk of recurrence due to the presence of scar tissue. This is prone to breakdown as it is physically weaker than the surrounding normal skin. Any early signs of pressure damage (*Table 2.3*) need to be recognised, and nursing strategies implemented to prevent deterioration.

❖ Impaired macro/micro-circulation

The skin as an organ only stays intact while it has sufficient blood supply, which may be affected by cerebro-vascular accident (CVA), peripheral vascular disease, neuropathy or hypoxia. When the micro-circulation to an area is impaired, it may be seen on the body as erythema or reactive hyperaemia (Russell, 2002) (*Table 2.3*).

❖ Sensitivity to pain or discomfort

Following a stroke or any disease process affecting the nerves, patients may not be aware of pain or discomfort which may lead to tissue damage and the subsequent development of superficial pressure ulcers. However, patients in pain may become immobile or may move frequently to ameliorate the pain. In each case, there may be an impact on skin integrity.

❖ Diabetes

Patients with diabetes are at a greater risk of the development of superficial pressure ulcers and poor wound healing (Silhi, 1998), particularly if blood glucose levels are poorly controlled. Lyder (2003) proposes that the effect of diabetes on the micro-circulation may be the reason for its predisposition to pressure ulcers. All patients who present with pressure ulceration should be screened for diabetes.

Extrinsic factors

❖ Patient mobility

Immobility is the most important factor in the development of pressure ulcers (Clay, 2000), which may occur within six hours (Lyder, 2003). Patient movement in bed, with the patient pushing on their heels, results in shear and friction, frequently leading to grade I and II pressure ulcers, commonly seen as blisters (Read, 2001).

❖ Nutritional status

Reduced fluid intake may lead to dehydration and dry skin. A patient's nutritional status can influence the development and treatment of a pressure ulcer (Royal College of Nursing [RCN], 2003; NICE, 2003). Approximately 40% of patients admitted into hospital have protein-energy malnutrition (PEM), likely to deteriorate during their stay (McWhirter and Pennington, 1994). Effects of malnutrition are observed as loss of muscle mass, loss of weight, impaired immunity, delayed wound healing, increased risk of complications and increased hospital stay (King's Fund Report, 1992). Weight loss can lead to loss of padding over bony prominences. Russell (2002) observes that: 'nutritional deficiencies can influence the development of a wound and also impair wound healing'. Conversely, the bariatric patient also presents with a high risk of pressure damage. Each patient has individual requirements which need regular assessment (Detsky and Baker, 1987; Deleany, 1990; Russell, 2002).

❖ Acute illness

A raised temperature associated with acute illness increases the risk of developing a superficial pressure ulcer (Jiricka *et al*, 1995). This has implications in both primary and secondary care, and could be a significant factor in the development of pressure ulcers in those that are already at risk.

Prevention of superficial pressure ulcers is both essential and desirable, and knowledge of the reasons why a person might develop superficial pressure damage is important (NICE, 2003, 2005).

Skin assessment and care

Skin inspection is necessary to provide baseline data and information on the effectiveness of any preventative plan (Dealey, 1999). Maintaining good skin condition can minimise skin breakdown (Dealey, 1999; Culley, 2002) and the development of superficial pressure ulcers. The pH of normal skin is 4–6.8 and this slight acidity contributes to its natural antibacterial properties. The state of the skin will be influenced by extremes of temperature, including the cold, sun exposure, smoking, air conditioning, and exposure to irritants and bacteria.

Skin inspection should occur regularly with the frequency being determined by changes in the patient's condition in relation to either deterioration or recovery (NICE, 2001a, b). Patients and carers should be taught how to monitor skin and be aware of the importance of reporting any changes. This is particularly important in the primary care environment, where healthcare professionals may spend only a limited time with the patient, the major care being provided by non-professional staff and carers.

Dealey (1999) suggests that assessment should include the following, and that skin assessment and skin changes should be recorded immediately (Nursing and Midwifery Council [NMC], 2002). Assessment of the skin overlying bony prominences should include:

- back of head
- shoulders
- elbows
- femoral trochanters
- ischial tuberosities
- sacrum
- heels
- toes.

Heels and elbows are particularly susceptible to tissue damage owing to the thin layer of subcutaneous tissue between skin and bone (Read, 2001; Black, 2004).

Skin status should be determined by identifying purplish/bluish patches on pigmented skin, red patches on light skin, swellings, blisters, shiny areas, dry patches and cracks, calluses and wrinkles. Signs to feel for are hard areas, warm areas, and swollen skin over bony points (NICE, 2001a, b). Areas prone to superficial pressure damage include heels, sacrum, ischial tuberosities and femoral trochanters.

When temporary occlusion of blood vessels occurs, the release of pressure produces a large and sudden increase in blood flow and this bright red flush is known as reactive hyperaemia (Morison, 2001; NICE, 2003). It is more difficult to assess in those with pigmented skin.

❖ 'Blanching hyperaemia is an area of erythema that turns white under finger pressure. When a bony prominence compresses the skin tissues against a hard surface (ie. the ischial tuberositites when in a seated position) the local blood supply will almost certainly be occluded and this leads to a blanching of the tissues. When the pressure is removed from the area, the capillaries over-react and flush bright red. This is known as reactive hyperaemia and is a healthy counteraction to the original occlusion. At this point, there is no lasting damage to the capillaries or to local tissues. Blanching hyperaemia could be used as a warning sign of patient risk. If the blanching redness does not fade within a few minutes, then it is important to consider a higher-grade mattress for this patient. When ignored, blanching hyperaemia can progress to tissue damage. Blanching hyperaemia is difficult to detect in dark or tanned skin' (Collins *et al*, 2002).

❖ 'Non-blanching erythema is a reddened area of the skin, which does not turn white under finger pressure. This indicates that damage has occurred due to unrelieved pressure and that inflammatory changes are present in the tissues. The patient requires immediate intervention, such as pressure-reducing equipment, increased frequency of mobilisation and repositioning schedules. Blanching hyperaemia is difficult to detect in dark or tanned skin, and physical assessment become important in reviewing risk in these patients, eg. heat over the area, solid or hardened tissue, darkened area of tissue' (Collins *et al*, 2002).

Assessment of superficial pressure ulcers

A careful examination of the superficial pressure ulcer and surrounding skin should be undertaken. The pressure ulcer should be classified using a recognised classification tool such as the NPUAP (1989, *Table 2.3*) or the EPUAP Guideline (EPUAP, 1999). Patients should receive an initial assessment in the first episode of care (within six hours) and ongoing risk assessment (NICE, 2005; NMPDU, 2002, 2005).

The areas to be examined include:

- site
- extent of non-blanchable erythema
- extent of broken skin damage
- wound measurement
- classification of the wound
- pain.

Table 2.3: Classification of NPUAP	
Grade I NPUAP	Grade II NPUAP
❖ Non-blanchable erythema of intact skin is seldom considered to be reversible	❖ Partial thickness skin loss involving epidermis and/or dermis
❖ Skin does not blanche, but may feel 'boggy' when compressed with a finger	❖ Tissue breaks down due to hypoxia and cell death
❖ Burst blood vessels result in extravasation of fluid into the tissues. This leads to swelling oedema which may precipitate distortion and thickening of tissues compressed between bone and a support surface	
❖ Discolouration can be red, dark red or purple	
❖ Early changes may not be seen in those with pigmented skin	

Management of superficial pressure ulcers

The management of superficial pressure ulcers requires interventions to prevent deterioration, and care to reduce the negative influences on the skin such as pressure, incontinence, reduced mobility/immobility, poor nutrition, abnormal body mass index (BMI), poor general skin condition and inadequate diet.

The treatment of superficial pressure ulcers is not an exact science and a multi-faceted approach is needed. This should include; the impact on quality of life, skin care, wound management, management of local and environmental issues, support surfaces, cushions, advice to patient and carers, psychological, social and spiritual support. Complex organisational approaches to prevention and treatment of superficial pressure ulcers should be considered, accommodating both local and national guidelines.

The success of wound healing depends on many intrinsic and extrinsic factors, eg. underlying disease, nutrition, and psychological well-being. To create a healing environment, all factors that adversely affect the health of the patient should be identified and, where possible, rectified. The wound should be classified, the surrounding skin assessed, and the assessment and management of pain undertaken (Stephen-Haynes and Gibson, 2003). Inadequate assessment, ie. the failure to address all the appropriate aspects of the patient's condition, or, the failure to assess at the optimum frequency, can lead to inappropriate wound management.

Impact on quality of life

Pressure ulcer prevention is an essential element of health care. It is important within all healthcare environments that there is a clear strategy about pressure ulcer prevention and treatment, which both needs to reflect national policies (Department of Health [DoH], 2001; NICE, 2001, 2003; NMPDU, 2002, 2005; RCN, 2003), and to be supported by management.

Far less research is undertaken on superficial pressure ulcers and their impact on the patient than on deep pressure ulcers. However, the progression from superficial to deep pressure ulcer can be rapid and strategies to prevent this from happening are essential.

Pressure ulcers damage not just the skin, but also the fatty tissue below, resulting in pain, extended hospitalisation and lengthy treatment. The deeper ulcers can also become infected, sometimes causing septicaemia and osteomyelitis. In severe cases, the underlying muscle or bone may be destroyed and, in extreme cases, pressure ulcers can become life-threatening (NICE, 2001b). While tissue damage is individual to every patient and their particular circumstances, pressure ulcers are considered to be an indicator of the quality of care provided by a hospital or unit. A phenomenological study (Fox, 2002) highlights the knowledge that deep pressure ulcers can be detrimental to patients with physical, psychological and social issues impacting on the patient in terms of suffering, loss of independence and mortality. Dealey (1999) similarly found all pressure ulcers to be detrimental to health and, significantly, observed the impact of pain, which led to the reduction of patient repositioning. As the anatomy and physiology would indicate, a superficial pressure ulcer with the exposure of nerves can be extremely painful. There are clearly implications when providing care for patients with superficial pressure ulcers of controlling pain, maintaining their ability to reposition, and preventing any further deterioration.

Positioning/repositioning

There is a significant link between the movem[...]
prevalence of pressure damage. Maylor (2004) [...]
as a means of redistributing pressure and redu[...]
advocate that patients who are at risk of pres[...]
should be repositioned, and the frequency of repositioning determined
by the results of skin inspection and individual needs, not by a ritualistic
schedule. The recommendations by NICE (2003) include:

- ❖ Repositioning should consider the patient's medical condition, their comfort, the overall plan of care and the support surface.
- ❖ Patients who are considered to be acutely at risk of developing pressure ulcers should be restricted to less than two hours of chair-sitting until their general condition improves.
- ❖ Positioning of patients should ensure that prolonged pressure on bony prominences is minimised, that bony prominences are kept from direct contact with one another, and that friction and shear damage is minimised. This may be achieved with pillows and foam pads.
- ❖ A repositioning schedule, agreed with the patient, should be recorded and established for each patient 'at risk'.
- ❖ Patients who are willing and able should be taught how to redistribute weight, with those in wheelchairs observing their skin using a mirror.
- ❖ Manual handling devices should be used correctly to minimise shear and friction damage. After manoeuvring, slings or other parts of the handling equipment should not be left underneath the patient.

Patients can be repositioned using the 30° tilt (Preston, 1984); however, there are no large clinical trials to support this approach and the importance appears to be repositioning whichever method is used. Conversely, Hampton (2001a) highlights the effective use of the 30° tilt in the prevention and treatment of pressure ulcers in South Africa where there is a lack of any pressure-reducing/relieving equipment.

dressings

osker et al (2005) identify many wound dressings available in the UK. Modern interactive dressings are recommended in the NICE draft guidelines on pressure ulcer treatment (NICE, 2005). While the lack of evidence is recognised by Morgan (2004), the practitioner should consider the following:

- appropriate size of dressing
- availability
- ease of application and removal
- maintaining the skin integrity: 'skin-friendly'
- avoidance of maceration
- comfort
- frequency of dressing changes.

Superficial pressure ulcers may be extremely painful and unlikely to produce large amounts of exudate. The key dressings for the management of these ulcers are barrier films, moisturising products, foam dressings, and, where there is exudate, hydrocolloid dressings.

Film dressings can act as an extra, protective layer, while allowing the skin to be observed. They must not be applied under tension as blistering of the skin may occur. The shiny surface may also be useful in reducing friction. Careful removal using a 'lateral stretching' technique is essential in preventing epidermal stripping. An area of redness can be outlined with a marker pen and clear acetate sheet in order to monitor progress. It is not suitable for moderate or heavy exudate as this can lead to maceration.

Hydrocolloids provide a moist environment and may be useful in autolytic debridement. The development of beveled-edged hydrocolloids assists in keeping them in place. Caution is needed with heavy exudate, and close monitoring is necessary for patients with wound infections.

Foam dressings offer comfort, absorbency and thermal insulation. They should be avoided in dry wounds. Alginates/Hydrofiber® are highly absorbent, form a gel with exudate and can be irrigated from a wound. They should be avoided in dry or lightly exuding wounds. Silicone dressings are considered as 'atraumatic' dressings. They are conformable and mouldable and easily removed. Hydrogels rehydrate and promote autolysis and may be left in place for one to three days. They should be avoided in heavily exuding wounds.

Any nurse prescribing needs to have a sound knowledge base and be able to provide a rationale for choice (Stephen-Haynes and Gibson, 2003). The prescribing nurse is legally responsible for ensuring that the product is used according to the manufacturer's instructions; this is particularly relevant in wound care products even when this duty has been delegated to another (Courtney and Butler, 1999). Further information is available at: www.dressings.org.

Pressure-relieving/reducing equipment

Pressure-relieving equipment has traditionally been identified as either pressure-reducing or pressure-relieving. Within the NICE (2003) guideline, they are all classified as 'pressure-relieving'. They have usefully been distinguished as 'low-tech' conforming mattresses, that distribute the body weight over a large area, and 'high-tech' alternating support surfaces, where cells alternately inflate and deflate (Cullum *et al*, 2001). The equipment has the aim of preventing the occurrence of superficial pressure damage, promoting healing of pressure ulcers, and promoting patient comfort (Cullum *et al*, 1995; Maylor, 2001; NICE, 2003). There is a lack of research on the efficacy and cost benefits of pressure-reducing/relieving equipment (Clark, 2004a), with both clinicians and managers questioning whether current allocations of equipment and budget are justifiable. Nevertheless, NICE (2003) offer guidance on equipment selection based upon expert opinion (*Table 2.4*). All who are vulnerable to pressure ulceration should, as a minimum, be placed on a high specification foam mattress (NICE, 2005).

Any equipment used will not negate the need for risk management, but form part of the overall care. Correct positioning, turning and transferring techniques are important to alleviate pressure and shear forces, and to encourage redistribution of weight on support surfaces. In summary, Maylor (2001) highlighted that equipment does not replace nursing care, but rather serves as an adjunct to care.

Pressure-redistributing equipment

Pressure-reducing equipment, also referred to as pressure-redistributing, is used widely in the advanced healthcare system (Gray *et al*, 1998; Maylor, 2001; Morison, 2001). High specification foam mattresses maximise the area of the patient's body in contact with the mattress surface, thereby reducing the extent of the interface pressure at any given anatomical location. Maylor (2001) notes that a standard hospital mattress provides an interface pressure of 145mmHg at the heel and 88mmHg at the sacrum, both of which are in excess of normal capillary closure pressure.

Table 2.4: Equipment selection	
Pressure-relieving devices: high-tech	Pressure-redistributing devices: low-tech
Dynamic alternating mattress replacement systems	Dynamic low air loss mattress replacement systems
Dynamic alternating mattress overlays	Dynamic low air loss mattress overlays
Dynamic alternating cushions	Gel mattresses
	Static foam mattresses
	Static foam overlays
	Static foam cushions

The use of a standard hospital mattress was identified as increasing the risk of the patient developing a pressure ulcer (Dealey, 1999). Cullum *et al* (1995) identify six randomised controlled studies and advocate high specification foam over the use of standard hospital foam mattresses for 'at risk' patients. This is similarly reiterated in the national guidelines (NICE, 2003), which propose that those at risk should, as a minimum, be provided with a high specification foam mattress with pressure-relieving properties. Bain *et al* (2004) undertook an evaluation of pressure-reducing mattresses on behalf of the Medical and Healthcare Products Regulatory agency (MHRA), exploring interface pressures, vapour transfer properties, fatigue longevity, fire retardency and mattress turning requirement. This highlights the significant difference between a NHS economy mattress and other pressure-reducing mattresses available. If pressure-redistributing mattresses are promptly provided before, or at the first sign of reddening, the patient is unlikely to develop a pressure ulcer (Hampton, 2001b). Maylor (2001) suggests that most of the evidence for the use of pressure-redistributing mattresses is derived from case studies or evaluations, not controlled trials. There are a number of high profile professionals who have advocated various pieces of equipment. Price *et al* (1999), in a small-scale study, found the Repose mattress (Frontier Therapeutics) prevented the development of pressure ulcers. Maylor (2001) notes the benefit of Roho dry flotation (Shiloh Healthcare) in pressure ulcer prevention, and this is reiterated within Worcestershire Primary Care Trust who have used them successfully in the prevention and treatment of superficial pressure ulcers for ten years. Hampton (1999), Russell (1999), and Gray *et al* (2000) found a benefit from visco-elastic foam in the prevention of pressure ulcers. However, Maylor (2001) noted that during a mattress evaluation, staff provided more preventative care to those with superficial pressure (grade I) ulcers, than those whose skin was intact.

Pressure-relieving systems

Cyclical alternating dynamic systems create a continuously changing interface pressure, usually to extremely low levels, independent of patient movement. This may be important because both the duration and intensity of pressure can influence the development and treatment of pressure ulcers. However, NICE (2003) conclude that there is insufficient evidence to support high-tech pressure-relieving devices over the low-tech foam mattresses. Important areas to consider are the level of risk, a twenty-four-hour approach, and the patient's previous history of pressure ulceration — their clinical condition indicates whether a high-tech device is necessary or where a low-tech piece has failed. Hampton and Collins (2004) emphasise the myth that patients on an air mattress do not need repositioning. Repositioning is necessary to reduce joint stiffness, improve breathing and mental status, irrespective of the support surface.

Cyclical replacements/overlays

Cyclical alternating dynamic systems come in two categories: pressure-relieving overlay mattresses and pressure-relieving replacement mattresses.

Overlay systems should be placed on top of the base mattress, while replacement mattresses should be placed directly on the bed without the base mattress. The cycles vary in speed and the number of cells which alternate.

NICE (2003) recommend that the pressure-relieving/reducing equipment choice should be based upon a full holistic assessment, including:

- level of risk
- skin assessment
- comfort
- general health status
- lifestyle and abilities
- critical care needs
- the twenty-four-hour period of care.

Other practical areas for consideration may include:

- quality of the product
- ability to profile
- repositioning
- reasonable weight for moving around
- patient's weight
- support of the patient's independent functioning
- cost of the product
- removable two-way stretch moisture vapour permeable cover
- meeting infection control requirements
- evidence to support product claims
- quality of after-service by manufacturer
- equipment tracking and management information
- technical service response
- user-friendliness of the product
- training and education required to use the product
- ease of use.

The following should **not** be used as pressure-relieving aids as they do not relieve pressure (NICE, 2001):

- water-filled gloves
- synthetic sheepskins (natural sheepskin may be effective in pressure ulcer prevention [NICE, 2003])
- doughnut-type devices.

Seating

Seating assessments for aids and equipment should be carried out by trained assessors who have the specific knowledge and expertise, eg. physiotherapists and occupational therapists. Advice should also be sought from trained assessors regarding correct seating position. Body weight, shear, friction, pelvic obliquity, lumbar lordosis and length of time sitting out, all influence the development of pressure ulcers. Particular care should be taken with those who are permanently seated, and whose body weight is supported by 8% of the seated area, predominantly around the ischial tuberosities (Wall and Colley, 2004). It is important that 'vulnerable patients' should be encouraged to go back to bed, rather than sit for long periods in a chair (Gebhardt and Bliss, 1994). In the UK, any wheelchair user with pressure-relieving requirement is entitled to be assessed for, and provided with, a suitable cushion or seating system (Collins, 2001a).

No seating cushion has been shown to perform better than another (NICE, 2001a; 2003), but consideration should be given to seating as part of the twenty-four-hour care plan. Cushions should provide the following (Collins, 2001b):

- maximum stability
- reduction in interface pressures over bony prominences
- stability for the pelvis
- comfort
- reduction in postural changes.

The advice of a seating therapist and access to a seating pressure monitor may be necessary. Specific patient groups, such as paediatric, obstetric, and bariatric have specific needs.

Monitoring pressure ulcers

It is the responsibility of every nurse, midwife and health visitor to strive for quality improvements in all aspects of practice (DoH, 1999). Pressure damage prevention, as previously mentioned, is seen as a quality indicator (DoH, 1992; 1999). Areas that an audit may include have been identified by NICE (2003), and an implementation guide has been developed which is designed to improve the quality of care for people at risk of developing pressure ulcers (RCN, 2003). The collection of such data is not mandatory.

Patient education

While there is a lack of high-grade research into the area of pressure ulcers (Clark, 2004b), care should be provided by staff that have received education and training. Staff levels, both in competence and numbers, need to reflect the needs of the patient. Continued education is imperative in preventing pressure ulcers in the future, and this is the responsibility of all staff. Patients need to be empowered and encouraged to take an active role in pressure ulcer prevention. The prevention of superficial pressure ulcers needs to be part of a comprehensive educational package that meets the needs of practitioners and patients.

Lloyd-Jones *et al* (2003) highlighted the need for education and training in an acute district general hospital. Audit had highlighted deficiencies in the knowledge base of staff and in the care given to prevent and manage pressure ulceration. Knowledge and understanding are major factors in compliance with treatment regimes. With physical recovery comes a lessening of the close observation and nursing attention. Verbal education should be reinforced by written information. Patients and, where appropriate, carers, who are able and willing, should be informed and educated about risk assessment and resulting prevention strategies. Patient/carer education, as recommended by NICE (2001b), should include information on the following :

- the risk factors associated with their developing pressure ulcers
- the sites that are at the greatest risk of pressure damage
- how to inspect skin and recognise skin changes
- where to seek further advice/assistance should they need it
- emphasis on the need for immediate referral to a healthcare professional should signs of skin damage be noticed.

Clinical benchmarking

The *Essence of Care* (DoH, 2001) provides clear patient-focused benchmarks on core and essential aspects of care to help improve quality. These benchmarks support the clinical governance agenda as set out in *A First Class Service* (DoH, 1999) and forms part of the NHS plan of improving the fundamentals and the patient experience of the Health Service. One of the benchmarks relates to pressure ulcer prevention. Benchmarking provides a useful tool for practitioners to take a structured approach to sharing and comparing practice, which enables them to identify best practice and develop action plans to improve quality (Culley, 2002; Butcher, 2004).

The nine factors identified in clinical benchmarking and pressure ulcer prevention are (DoH, 2001):

- screening/assessment
- who undertakes the assessment
- informing patients/clients/carers (prevention and treatment)
- individualised plan for prevention and treatment of pressure ulcers
- pressure ulcer prevention — repositioning
- pressure ulcer prevention — redistributing support surfaces
- pressure ulcer prevention — availability of resources, equipment
- implementation of individualised plan
- evaluation of interventions by registered practitioner.

Accountability

The Nursing and Midwifery Council (NMC, 2002) identifies the professional's accountability for providing care, and also explicitly communicating with patients, carers and members of the healthcare team. It is essential that risk factors are identified, documented, reviewed and acted upon. This needs to be seen as a continual process as evidence suggests that while we undertake initial assessments, we are generally poorer at re-assessment (Russell, 2003). With increased autonomy comes an increase in accountability. And, as accountable professionals, nurses must be able to explain and justify why they make decisions. All nurses need to know to whom they are accountable:

- the NMC
- the public
- the patient
- the employer.

A thorough knowledge of accountability and its implications for practice will ensure that nurses continue to develop their practice in response to patient and professional need, in a safe and competent way (Glover, 1999). The NMC defines accountability as 'an integral part of nursing practice'. To be accountable, the practitioner must be guided by research-based standards.

Conclusion

With the recent publication of the consolidated Nice guideline on pressure ulcer management and treatment, healthcare professionals have been provided with the evidence base to support their arguments to implement measures to prevent and best manage superficial pressure ulcers. With increased autonomy comes an increase in accountability, and as accountable professionals, nurses must be able to explain and justify the decisions that they make. Superficial pressure ulcers pose a significant challenge to patients, carers and healthcare practitioners. Identifying superficial pressure ulcers is a significant aspect of assessment and planning treatment, and international concensus will assist this. It is important for healthcare practitioners to have education of pathophysiology, skin assessment, skin care, selection of pressure-relieving equipment, repositioning, national guidelines and audit. Prevention of pressure damage is essential and, where superficial pressure damage does exist, it is important to prevent any further deterioration.

References

Bain D, Ferguson-Pell M, Nicholson G (2004) Pressure reducing mattresses. MHRA Evaluation. 03129-0 and03129 April. Available online at: nww.medical-devices.nhs.uk

Bennett L, Lee B (1985) Pressure versus sheer in pressure sore formation. In: Lee B, ed. *Chronic Ulcers of the Skin*. McGraw-Hill, London

Black J (2004) *Preventing Heel Pressure Ulcers*. Lippincott Williams and Wilkins Inc, London

Bridel J (1993) The aetiology of pressure sores. *J Wound Care* **2**(4): 230–8

Butcher M (2002) Barrier for effective wound care. Presented at 9th European conference on Advances in Wound Management, Harrogate, UK

Butcher M (2004) *NICE Guidelines: Pressure ulcer risk assessment and prevention — a review*. Available online at: http://wwwworldwidewounds.com

Clark M (1996) The aetiology of superficial sacral pressure sores. In: Leaper DL, Cherry GW, Dealey C, eds. Proceedings of the 6th European Conference on Advances in Wound Management, Amsterdam. Macmillan Press: 167–9

Clark M (2004a) Barriers to the implementation of clinical guidelines. In: White R, ed. *Trends in Wound Care, volume III*. Quay Books, MA Healthcare Ltd, London

Clark M (2004b) *Pressure Ulcers: Recent advances in tissue viability*. Quay Books, MA Healthcare Ltd, London

Clay M (2000) Pressure sore prevention in nursing homes. *Nurs Standard* **1**(44): 45–50

Clever K, Smith G, Bowser C, Monroe K (2002) Evaluating the efficacy of a uniquely delivered protectant and its effect on the formation of sacral/ buttock pressure ulcers. *Ostomy Wound Management* **48**(912): 60–7

Collins F (2001a) How to assess a patient's seating needs: some basic principles. *J Wound Care* **10**(9): 383–6

Collins F (2001b) *Seating*. Educational leaflet no 8. Wound Care Society, Huntingdon: 1–7

Collins F (2002) Use of pressure reducing seats and cushions in a community setting. *Br J Community Nurs* **7**(1): 15–22

Collins F, Hampton S, White R (2004) *A–Z Dictionary of Wound Care*. Quay Books, MA Healthcare Ltd, London

Cosker T, Elsayed S, Gupta S *et al* (2005) Choice of dressings has a major impact on blistering and healing outcomes. *J Wound Care* **14**(1): 27–9

Courtney M, Butler M (1998) *Nurse Prescribing Principles and Practice*. Grenwich Medical Media, London: 1–5

Culley F (2002) Nursing aspects of pressure ulcer prevention and therapy. In: White R, ed. *Trends in Wound Care, volume I*. Quay Books, MA Healthcare Ltd, London

Cullum N, Deeks J, Fletcher A, Shelton T (1995) The prevention and treatment of pressure sores: how effective are pressure relieving interventions and risk assessment for the prevention and treatment of pressure sores? Effective Health Care Bulletin. NHS Centres for Reviews and Dissemination. University of York, York

Cullum N, Nelson E, Fleming K, Sheldon T (2001) Systematic reviews of wound care management. (5) Beds Health Technology Assessment (HTA), National Coordinating Centre for Health Technology Assessment (NCCHTA), University of Southampton

Dealey C (1999) *The Care of Wounds: A guide for nurses*. Blackwell Scientific Publication, Oxford

Deleany HM (1990) Effects of early post-operative nutritional support on skin wound and colon anastomosis healing. *J Parental Enteral Nutrition* **140**: 357–61

Department of Health (1992) *The Health of the Nation: A strategy for health in England*. HMSO, London.

Department of Health (1999) *Making a Difference: A strategy for nursing*. DoH, London

Department of Health (1999) *NHS Plan: A first class service*. DoH, London

Depatment of Health (2001) *The Essence of Care: Patient-focused benchmarking for health care practitioners*. DoH, London

Detsky AS, Baker JP (1987) Perioperative nutrition: a meta-analysis of the literature. *Ann Intern Med* **107**: 195–203

European Pressure Ulcer Advisory Panel (1999) Guidelines on treatment of pressure ulcers. *EPUAP Review* **1**(2): 136–69

Fox C (2002) Living with a pressure ulcer: a descriptive study of patients' experiences. Wound Care. *Br J Community Nurs*: **7**(6) S10–S22

Glover D (1999) *Accountability — Monographs*. Nurs Times. Emap Healthcare Ltd, London

Gray D, Cooper P, Campbell M (1998) A study of the performance of a pressure reducing foam mattress after 3 years of use. *J Tissue Viability* **8**(3): 9–13

Gray D, Whelan S, Russell G et al (2000) Evaluation of an electric bed frame and pressure reducing mattress. *Br J Community Nurs* **5**(12): 596–602

Hampton S (1999) Efficacy and cost effectiveness of the Thermo-contour mattress. *Br J Nurs* **8**(15): 990–6

Hampton S (2001a) Pressure ulcer care: can we learn from poorer countries? *Br J Nurs* **10**(6): S4

Hampton S (2001b) Equipment to prevent pressure ulcers in low risk residents. *Nurs Residential Care* **3**(2): 72–5

Hampton S (2002) Introducing the reflexion pressure redistributing cushion. *Br J Nurs* **11**(7): 509–13

Hampton S, Collins F (2004) *Tissue Viability. The prevention, treatment and management of wounds*. Whurr Publishers, London

Jiricka MK, Ryan P, Carvalho MA, Bukvitch J (1995) Pressure ulcer risk factors in an ICU population. *Am J Crit Care* **4**(5): 361–7

Lewis-Byers K, Thayer D, Khal A (2002) An evaluation of two incontinence skincare protocols in a long-term care setting. *Ostomy Wound Management* **48**(12): 44–51

Lyder C (2003) Pressure ulcer prevention and management. *JAMA* **289**(2): 223–6

Lloyd-Jones M, Young T, Liptrot P (2003) Improving pressure ulcer care through designer education. *Br J Nurs* (Tissue Viability Supplement) **12**(19): S28–S32

King's Fund Report (1992) *A Positive Approach to Nutrition as Treatment.* King's Fund, London

Maylor M (2001) Pressure reducing equipment 3: static systems. *Nurs Residential Care* **3**(11): 522–9

Maylor M (2004) Manual repositioning: turning patients and reducing risk.In Clark M, ed. *Pressure Ulcers: Recent advances in tissue viability.* Quay Books, MA Healthcare Ltd, London

McWhirter JP, Pennington CR (1994) Incidence and recognition of malnutrition in hospital. *Br Med J* **308**(6934): 945–8

Morison M *et al* (2001) *The Prevention and Treatment of Pressure Ulcers.* Mosby, London

National Institute for Clinical Excellence (NICE) (2001a) *Pressure Ulcer Risk Assessment and Prevention — Inherited Clinical Guideline B.* NICE, London. Available online at: http://www. nice.org.uk

National Institute for Clinical Excellence (NICE) (2001b) *Pressure Ulcer Risk Assessment and Prevention. A guide for patients and their carers.* NICE, London. Available online at: http://www. nice.org.uk

National Institute for Clinical Excellence (NICE) (2003) *Pressure Ulcer Risk Assessment and Prevention and Equipment Selection.* NICE, London. Available online at: http://www. nice.org.uk

National Institute for Clinical Excellence (NICE) (2005) *Pressure ulcers: the management of pressure ulcers in primary and secondary care.* (Draft) NICE, London. Available online at: http://www. nice.org.uk

National Pressure Ulcer Advisory Panel (1989) Incidence, economics and risk assessment. *Care Sci Practice* **7**(4): 96–9

Nursing and Midwifery Council (2002) *Code of Professional Conduct.* NMC, London

Nursing and Midwifery Practice Development Unit (2002) Pressure Ulcer Prevention: Best Practice Statement. NMPDU, Edinburgh. Available online at: http://www.nhshealthquality.org/nhsqis/files/BPSPressureUlcer Prevention.pdf

Nursing and Midwifery Practice Development Unit (2005) The Treatment/ management of Pressure Ulcers: Best Practice Statement. NMPDU, Edinburgh. Available online at: http://nhshealthquality.org/nhsqis/files/BPS %20Management%20Pressure%20Ulcers%20(Mar%202005).pdf

Preston K (1984) Positioning for comfort and pressure relief: the 30° alternative. *Care Sci Practice* **6**(4): 116–9

Price P, Bale S, Newcombe R (1999) Challenging the pressure sore paradigm. *J Wound Care* **8**(4): 180–90

Read S (2001) Treatment of a blister caused by pressure and friction. *Br J Nurs* **10**(1): 10–19

Royal College of Nursing (2000) *Clinical practice guidelines. Pressure ulcer risk assessment and prevention.* RCN, London

Royal College of Nursing (2003) *Pressure ulcer risk assessment and prevention. Implementation guide and protocol. Improving practice: improving care.* RCN, London

Russell L (1999) A review of the Medical Agency services Comfor-med range. *Br J Nurs* **8**(10): 681–6

Russell L (2002) The importance of patients' nutritional status in wound healing. In: White R, ed. *Trends in Wound Care, volume I.* Quay Books, MA Healthcare Ltd, London

Russell L (2003) Pressure ulcer classification: the systems and the pitfalls.In: White R, ed. *Trends in Wound Care, volume II.* Quay Books, MA Healthcare Ltd, London

Satsue H, Tatsuo S, Hiromi A, Yuji A (2005) Morphological architecture and distribution of blood capillaries and elastic fibres in the human skin. In: Clark M, ed. *Pressure Ulcers: Recent advances in tissue viability.* Quay Books, MA Healthcare Ltd, London

Schuren J, Becker A, Sibbald RG (2005) A liquid film-forming acrylate for peri-wound protection: a systematic review and meta-analysis (3M™ Cavilon™ No Sting Barrier film). *Int Wound J* **2**(3): 230–8

Silhi N (1998) Diabetes and wound healing. *J Wound Care* **7**: 47–51

Stephen-Haynes J, Gibson E (2003) *Anatomy, Physiology and Wound Assessment.* Wound Care Society, Huntingdon

Touche Ross (1993) *The Cost of Pressure Sores.* DoH/Touche Ross, London

Waterlow J (1985) Pressure sores: a risk assessment card. *Nurs Times* **81**(48): 49–95

Versluysen M (1986) How elderly patients develop pressure ulcers in hospital. *Br Med J* **292**: 1311–13

Wall J, Colley T (2004) Preventing pressure ulcers among wheelchair users: preliminary comments on the development of a self-administered risk assessment tool. Available online at: http://worldwidewounds.com

CHAPTER 3

SUPERFICIAL DIABETIC FOOT ULCERS

Caroline McIntosh and Veronica Newton

To address the theme of superficial diabetic foot ulcers, it is pertinent to outline the extent of the challenge. Recent statistics suggest at least 1.3 million people in the UK have diagnosed type 2 diabetes, with an estimated further 600,000 to 800,000 undiagnosed (National Institute for Clinical Excellence [NICE], 2004).

The direct economic cost of diabetic foot ulcers to the healthcare system is high; the estimated cost for diabetic foot ulcer management is £1451 per case, or £17 million per year nationally (Currie, 1998). This does not measure the indirect costs of foot ulceration to the person with diabetes, which may have dramatic effects on physical, mental, and spiritual well-being.

In terms of the burden of foot problems among people with diabetes, complications in the foot are common, with 20%–40% of people estimated to have neuropathy, and about 5% a foot ulcer (Kumar *et al*, 1994; Walters *et al*, 1992; Neil *et al*, 1989). Therefore, healthcare professionals regularly involved in treating patients with diabetes will, undoubtedly, be involved in the management of foot ulceration.

It is critical that diabetic foot ulcers receive the best standard of care. The ten-year target of the *National Service Framework (NSF) for Diabetes* (Department of Health [DoH], 2001) requires healthcare practitioners to achieve its 12 standards by 2013. Standard 11 is particularly pertinent with respect to the chronic complications affecting the foot in relation to the aetiology of diabetic foot ulcers.

The NHS will develop, implement and monitor agreed protocols and systems of care to ensure that all people who develop long-term complications of diabetes receive timely, appropriate, and effective investigation and treatment to reduce their risk of disability and premature death.

Part I: Assessment

Identifying risk factors

Despite a wealth of evidence, the prevention of diabetic foot ulcers remains a significant challenge for practitioners involved in diabetes care. Yet, the majority of diabetes-related foot lesions remain largely preventable. Early identification, early recognition, and appropriate management of risk factors associated with diabetic foot ulceration can prevent adverse outcomes such as ulcer development.

Approximately 40%–60% of all non-traumatic lower leg amputations are performed in patients with diabetes (International Working Group on the Diabetic Foot, 1999), therefore, all healthcare practitioners involved in the care of diabetic patients must have an appreciation of the general factors associated with diabetic foot ulcers (*Box 3.1*).

Box 3.1: Factors associated with foot ulcers

❖ Previous ulcer.
❖ Neuropathy — sensorimotor.
❖ Trauma — footwear/walking barefoot.
❖ Biomechanics — limited joint mobility/foot deformity.
❖ Peripheral vascular disease.
❖ Socio-economic status — poor education and poor access to health care (social isolation).

(International Working Group on the Diabetic Foot, 1999)

It is widely recognised that the presence of peripheral neuropathy is a major contributory factor in the development of diabetic foot ulceration. This is often complicated by the presence of peripheral vascular disease (PVD). Diabetic neuropathy and the presence of PVD are associated with poor glycaemic control and factors associated with vascular disease (*Boxes* 3.2 and 3.3).

Box 3.2: Additional factors associated with foot ulcers

* Approximately 50% of people who present at diabetic foot clinics have neuropathy and 50% have neuroischaemic feet (Edmonds and Foster, 1999).
* Glycaemic control, ethnic background, duration of disease, and cardiovascular factors are all associated with increased risk of complications.

(NICE, 2004)

Diabetic peripheral neuropathy can affect sensory, motor and autonomic nerve pathways. *Box 3.4* outlines the effects of peripheral neuropathy in the lower limb.

Structural changes and foot deformity can develop secondary to peripheral neuropathy (*Box 3.5*).

The presence of PVD in patients with diabetes can prove limb-threatening; the majority of amputations preceded by foot ulceration are performed

Box 3.3: Risk factors associated with peripheral vascular disease

* Hypertension.
* Dyslipidaemia.
* Coronary heart disease.
* Smoking.
* Hyperglycaemia.
* Renal disease.

on ischaemic limbs. The duration of diabetes and the extent of hyperglycaemia correlate in randomised controlled trials (Diabetes Control and Complications Trial [DCCT], 1993; UK Prospective Diabetes Study [UKPDS], 1999), with the development of vascular complications distal to the popliteal vessels. Arterial pain, such as intermittent claudication, is often the first indicator of vessel disease in a non-diabetic patient, however, due to the presence of peripheral neuropathy, patients may remain asymptomatic. The practitioner should be extra vigilant in the care of the patient with neuroischaemic diabetes.

Box 3.4: Effect of peripheral neuropathy on the lower extremities

Sensory neuropathy	Motor neuropathy	Autonomic neuropathy
Loss of sensation plays a significant role in ulcer development. Ulcer risk is increased by 7-fold in the insensitive foot.

(Buchman, 2005) | Altered mechanics and foot deformity can result in abnormal plantar pressures which can increase ulceration risk.

(Abouaesha *et al*, 2001) | Decreased sweating and anhydrotic skin can result in callus formation under site-increased pressure. Anhydrotic skin is fragile and prone to fissuring, posing a risk for secondary infection.

(Abouaesha *et al*, 2001) |

Box 3.5: Common structural changes in the diabetic foot

* Clawed digits.
* Plantarflexion of the metatarsal heads.
* Anterior migration of fibrofatty padding.
* Limited joint mobility.
* *Pes cavus* (high medial longitudinal arch profile).

(Abouaesha *et al*, 2001)

Further reading and useful websites

Blood glucose management: http://www.nice.org.uk/pdf/NICE_full_blood_glucose.pdf

Blood pressure management: http://www.sheffield.ac.uk/guidelines/bpmanagement/bpmanagement.pdf

Boulton AJM, Connor H, Cavanagh PR *et al* (2000) *The Foot in Diabetes*. 2nd edn. Wiley, Chichester

Bowker JH, Pfiefer MA, eds (2001) *Levin and O'Neal's The Diabetic Foot*. 6th edn. Mosby, USA

UKPDS: http://www.dtu.ox.ac.uk/index.html?maindoc=/ukpds/

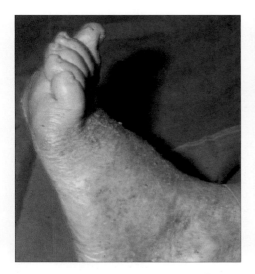

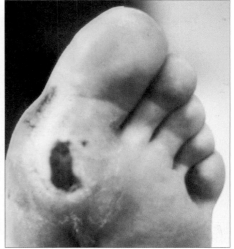

Figure 3.1: Common structural changes associated with motor neuropathy

Figure 3.2: Superficial diabetic foot ulceration on the plantar first metatarsophalangeal joint associated with high pressure in an insensitive foot

Assessment of the diabetic foot

All individuals with diabetes should receive annual assessment by trained personnel as part of ongoing care (NICE, 2004). NICE guidelines specify minimum requirements for basic foot examination (*Box 3.6*).

Following basic foot examination, risk status should be classified (*Box 3.7*) to ensure effective management of patients considered to be at greatest risk of ulceration.

Box 3.6: Basic foot examination

Examination of feet should include:
* Use of 10 gram monofilament to assess for sensory neuropathy.
* Palpation of foot pulses to detect significant changes in peripheral circulation.
* Inspection of the foot for deformities.
* Inspection of footwear for wear and tear and foreign objects that may traumatise the foot.

(NICE, 2004)

Box 3.7: Classification system

- ❖ Classify foot risk.
- ❖ Low risk (no complications) — annual review.
- ❖ At-risk foot (neuropathy or absent pulse or other) — 3/6-monthly review.
- ❖ High-risk foot (risk factor and deformity/previous ulcer) 1/3-monthly/individualised plan.
- ❖ Ulcerated foot — urgent treatment.

(Hutchinson *et al*, 2000)

Even in the presence of neuropathy or ischaemia, deterioration may be halted by tight control of blood glucose, blood pressure, lipids and smoking cessation (*Box 3.8*).

Box 3.8: Control of risk factors

The incidence of micro-vascular and macro-vascular endpoints of diabetes at increasing HbA_{1c} or systolic blood pressure levels show a linear relationship, indicating any reduction in glycaemia or blood pressure would be advantageous for the person with diabetes. The study data support previous guidelines and suggest patients should aim for near-normal levels, in practice aiming for targets for HbA_{1c}<7%, and blood pressure <140/<80mmHg.

(UKPDS, 1998)

Since HbA_{1c} measurement is a predictor of the rate of development of micro- and macro-vascular disease, a 2–6-monthly review is recommended.

(Hutchinson *et al*, 2000)

Further reading and useful websites

Edmonds M, Foster A (1999) _Managing the Diabetic Foot_. Blackwell Science, Oxford

International Working Group on the Diabetic Foot (1999) _International Consensus on the Diabetic Foot_. Amsterdam, The Netherlands

National Service Framework For Diabetes: Standards (Department of Health 2001)

National Service Framework For Diabetes: Delivery Strategy (Department Of Health 2002)

Diabetes UK: http://www.diabetes.org.uk/

National Institute of Clinical Excellence: http://www.nice.org.uk

RCGP Guidelines: http://www.sheffield.ac.uk/guidelines/guidelines/ footcare.pdf

Diabetes Competence Framework — Skills For Health Online Database: http://195.10.235.25/standards_database/index.htm

Dermatological assessment

The practitioner should assess the diabetic foot for any skin abnormalities, such as visible lesions and breaches in skin integrity. Interdigital spaces should be checked for signs of maceration, inflammation and digital pressure (ie. heloma molle [soft corns]), as these may be indicative of a pre-ulcerative state.

Figures 3.3 to _3.8_ illustrate common skin lesions that can result in breaches in skin integrity, infection and ulceration.

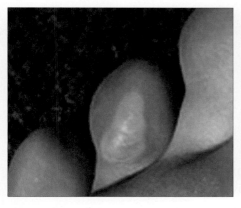

Figure 3.3: Blisters

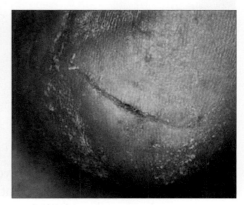

Figure 3.4: Fissures

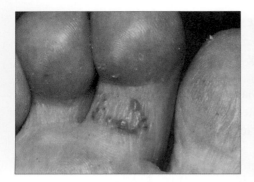

Figure 3.5: Fungal infections

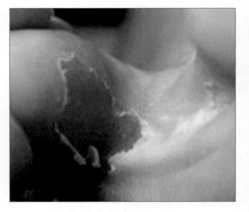

Figure 3.6: Interdigital maceration

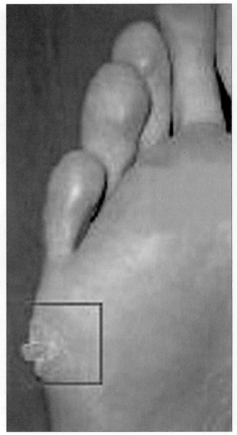

Figure 3.8: Callus

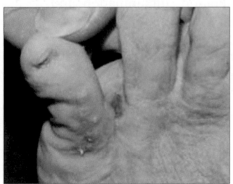

Figure 3.7: Corns (dorsal
and interdigital)

The following assessment framework is recommended to assist the
practitioner either at the pre-ulcerative stage, or, in the case of a newly-
presenting ulcer — the **ALERT** system.

A **Ask the patient** about the skin — how does it feel to them? By undertaking a thorough history and encouraging the patient to vocalise their concerns, clinical links can be made to diagnose the aetiology of skin changes (*Table 3.1*).

L **Look at the skin** — is it intact? By visually examining and scrutinising the surrounding tissues, practitioners can quickly develop an appreciation of the

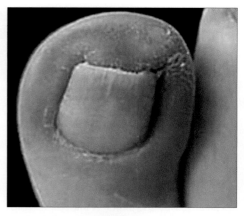

Figure 3.9: Cellulitis on the lateral aspect of the hallux

early signs of skin changes that may be indicative of pre-ulcerative stages or underlying complications (*Table 3.1*).

E **Examine** for signs of infection — heat, redness, pain, swelling, or look for any foot complications (*Figure 3.9*). Foot ulcers are susceptible to infection which may spread rapidly causing tissue destruction (Edmonds and Foster, 1999). This process is the main reason for major amputation in neuropathic feet.

R **Review** previous treatment and the patient's notes — this simple process may be the absolute key to the success of future management to discover any compliance/personal neglect issues, or to negotiate any changes needed to the management plan.

T **Think** about an individualised management plan — be practical and realistic: does your patient have the ability to access the health care? Consider transport, support networks, family/work commitments.

Skin changes in the diabetic foot

It is important that the healthcare practitioner has an appreciation of the changes that may occur in the skin associated with diabetes (*Table 3.1*).

There are several diabetes mellitus-specific conditions that dermatologists must be aware of, including, *necrobiosis lipoidica diabeticorum*, granuloma annulare, diabetic dermopathy (spotted leg syndrome or shin spots), diabetic bullae (*bullosis diabeticorum*), and waxy skin syndrome.

Table 3.1: Dermatological changes in diabetes		
Connective tissue skin changes	Neuropathic skin changes	Ischaemic skin changes
Dry skin	Dry skin	Dry skin
Inflexibility of tissues	Dilated veins	Atrophy of subcutaneous layer/thinning of skin
Limitation of joint mobility	Warm to touch	Cold to touch
Hardness to the skin texture	Pink/red in colour *(Figure 3.10)*	Cyanosed colour *(Figure 3.11)*
	Extravasated plantar callosities (spots of blood)	Hair loss

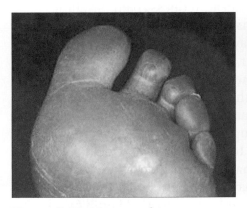

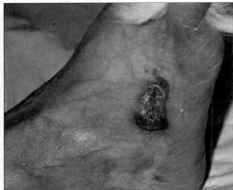

Figure 3.10: Neuropathic skin changes

Figure 3.11: Ischaemic skin changes

Part II: Prevention of diabetic foot ulceration

Regular assessment, prompt identification of risk factors, and the implementation of an appropriate management plan, can largely prevent ulcer formation. Published strategies for the prevention of ulceration are listed in *Box 3.9*.

Skin care

The diabetic foot should be regularly inspected for the presence of areas of high pressure. The formation of callus or corn is a positive indicator of high pressure, and is an independent risk factor for ulceration. There is evidence that the skilled debridement of such lesions decreases plantar pressure (Murray *et al*, 1996; Young *et al*, 1992). Careful assessment and, if necessary, debridement of such lesions is of paramount importance in the management and prevention of foot ulcers.

> ## Box 3.9: Strategies to prevent ulceration
>
> Published strategies for the prevention of ulceration include:
> ❖ Skin and nail care.
> ❖ Therapeutic footwear and insoles.
> ❖ Multidisciplinary foot care.
> ❖ Foot care education.
>
> (NICE, 2004; Maciejewski *et al*, 2004)

Haemorrhagic callus indicates high levels of pressure and forewarns of potential tissue breakdown. *Figures 3.12* and *3.13* illustrate haemorrhagic callus requiring sharp debridement.

Callus accentuates pressure and should be debrided to prevent tissue breakdown and/or allow the extent of any underlying ulceration to be evaluated. *Figures 3.16a* and *16b* (*p. 63*) show an area of haemorrhagic callus pre- and post-debridement. Following sharp debridement an area of ulceration is exposed.

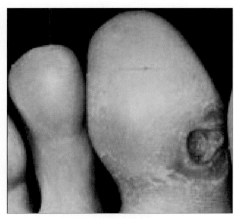

Figure 3.12: Haemorrhagic callus over the interphalangeal joint of the right hallux

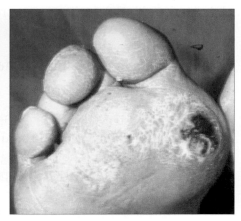

Figure 3.13: Haemorrhagic calluses over the first and fifth plantar metatarsal heads

Patients with diabetes presenting with skin or nail pathologies should receive prompt referral to podiatry for skilled debridement and regular palliative care. Data from randomised controlled trials studying the impact of podiatric care in the primary and secondary prevention of diabetic foot ulceration, suggest that regular palliative care of skin and nail pathologies results in a lower prevalence of ulceration and amputation for patients with diabetes (Plank *et al*, 2003; Ronnemaa *et al*, 1997).

Education

Since its publication in 2001, the *NSF for Diabetes* has contributed to the focus on structured education in an attempt to prevent some of the devastating complications associated with diabetes.

The NICE Health Technology Appraisal on patient-education models for diabetes, describes structured education as something which is a comprehensive, planned, graded and flexible programme that responds to an individual's clinical and psychological needs, within their educational and cultural background.

The primary goal for the diabetes care provider is to enable the patient living with diabetes to manage their own diabetes and foot care independently. The *NSF for Diabetes* recommends structured education to improve the patient's knowledge and understanding of their condition, enabling them to undertake effective self-care (DoH, 2005).

Foot care education is imperative in the prevention of diabetic foot ulceration. *Table* 3.2 outlines some recommendations for foot education.

Further reading and useful websites

Edmonds ME, Foster A, Sanders (2004) *A Practical Manual of Diabetic Footcare*. Blackwell Science, Oxford

Report from patient education working group: http://www.dh.gov.uk/assetRoot/04/11/31/97/04113197.pdf; http://www.dh.gov.uk/assetRoot/04/11/32/17/04113217.pdf

National Structured Education Programmes: http://www.dafne.uk.com/; www.desmond-project.org.uk

Table 3.2: Patient education

Daily foot inspections should be advised. If this is not feasible, encourage a family member or carer to undertake this role

Advice should be given on basic foot hygiene

Advise thorough drying between toes to reduce the risk of fungal infection

Regular emollient use can reduce anhydrosis and the formation of callus and fissuring of the skin

If the patient notices any breach in the skin, they should contact a member of the foot care team immediately

Hosiery should not be tight — elastic can impair circulation into the foot

Footwear should always be fitted to avoid pressure lesions from ill-fitting shoes

Diabetic patients should be advised to never walk barefoot, they should always wear protective footwear to avoid trauma

Any skin or nail pathologies should be managed by a podiatrist. Patients should be discouraged from undertaking self-care of pathological nails or skin lesions

Patients presenting with non-pathological toenails should be encouraged in safe self-care

Diabetic foot ulcers are not inevitable. With regular assessment, early detection of risk factors associated with ulceration, and prompt management, foot ulcers are largely preventable.

The following framework is recommended to assist the practitioner in the prevention of primary or secondary diabetic foot ulceration — the **PREVENT** system.

P **Palliative care** — regular palliative skin and nail care are required to reduce the likelihood of foot ulceration occurring secondary to nail or skin pathologies.

R **Regular risk assessment** should be undertaken by appropriately trained health professionals to identify factors that increase the risk of ulceration.

E **Educate the patient**.

V **Visual assessment** should be undertaken regularly by trained professionals to identify any skin lesions or nail pathologies that could compromise tissue viability in the diabetic foot.

E **Empower the patient** — Professionals should encourage patients living with diabetes to manage their own diabetes and foot health to the best of their ability.

N **Negotiate** an appropriate management plan with the patient and their carers, ensuring that the patient's needs are addressed.

T **Team approach** — refer patients at risk of foot ulceration to the multidisciplinary foot care team for assessment and on-going care.

Part III: Management of superficial diabetic foot ulcers

Wound classification

Dealey (2005) considers any breach in the continuity of the skin to be a wound. The aetiology of wounds in a patient with diabetes is often multifactoral. Abnormalities of the vascular and neurological systems make the diabetic foot susceptible to abnormal mechanical stresses that can lead to a breach in skin integrity. Once the skin barrier is broken, wound healing can be impaired by peripheral arterial disease and abnormally functioning white blood cells. The accompanying loss of protective sensation from neurological dysfunction prevents the patient perceiving intolerable loads being applied to the area and the common result is tissue failure and ulcer formation.

Classification systems (eg. [Meggitt] Wagner scale, Texas classification system) are frequently employed when attempting to quantify a wound. To make a classification system clinically relevant, it should be easy to use, reproducible, and effective to communicate wound status accurately.

Systematically recording the characteristics of ulcerations is critical to plan treatment strategies, monitor treatment effectiveness, predict clinical outcomes, and improve communication among healthcare providers. The most commonly cited diabetic wound classification system is the Wagner scale. The system is based mainly on wound depth and consists of six wound grades (*Table 3.3*).

Armstrong (1998) identifies that the Wagner scale is limited. It does not allow classification of superficial wounds affected by infection or PVD. A further limitation is that only the most severe signs of vascular disease (forefoot gangrene and whole foot gangrene) are considered.

The University of Texas wound classification system uses a system of wound grade and stage to categorise. Wounds are graded by depth: grade 0 represents a pre- or post-ulcerative site. Grade I ulcers are superficial wounds penetrating the epidermis and/or dermis but do not penetrate to tendon, capsule or bone. Grade II wounds penetrate to tendon or capsule. Grade III wounds penetrate to bone or into a joint. Within each wound grade there are four stages: (A) clean wounds; (B) non-ischaemic infected wounds; (C) ischaemic wounds; and (D) infected ischaemic wounds (*Table 3.4*).

Table 3.3: Wagner scale	
Grade 0	Intact skin
Grade I	Superficial ulcer
Grade II	Deep ulcer to tendon, bone or joint
Grade III	Deep ulcer with abscess or osteomyelitis
Grade IV	Forefoot gangrene
Grade V	Whole foot gangrene

Table 3.4: The University of Texas classification system				
Stage	**Grade**			
	0	**I**	**II**	**III**
A	Pre- or post-lesion intact	Superficial wound	Penetrating to tendon or capsule	Penetrating to bone or joint
B	+ infection	+ infection	+ infection	+ infection
C	+ ischaemia	+ ischaemia	+ ischaemia	+ ischaemia
D	+ infection and ischaemia	+ infection and ischaemia	+ infection and ischaemia	+ infection and ischaemia

For the purpose of this chapter, emphasis is placed on the management of superficial diabetic foot ulceration; ulcers considered to be grade I using the aforementioned classification systems.

Differences between neuropathic and ischaemic foot wounds

Neuropathic wounds

The clinical spectrum of neuropathy is complex in terms of presentation and progression, with patients developing sometimes large painless lesions — this is a major challenge for patients and practitioners alike (*Boxes 3.4* and *3.5*).

Ischaemic wounds

The manifestations of skin changes in the ischaemic foot are often demonstrated by the presence of painful ulcerations on the borders of the digits, aspices of the toes and dorsum of the foot.

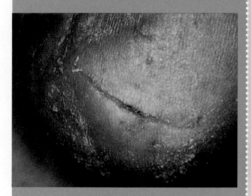

Figure 3.14: Superficial fissure on the plantar surface of a neuropathic heel which, if not treated promptly, can lead to secondary infection and ulceration at the site

Debridement is the removal of necrotic (dead) tissue by sharp surgical, chemical or other means, eg. larval therapy (*Box 3.12*).

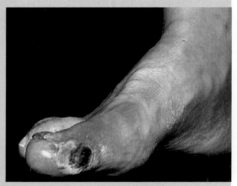

Figure 3.15: Ischaemic ulcer on the medial border of the right hallux caused by minor trauma, which is starting to develop signs of spreading cellulitis

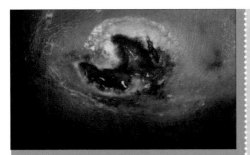

Figure 3.16a: Pre-debridement of a painless plantar lesion (note the extravasated callus)

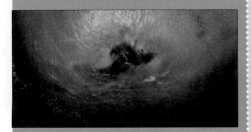

Figure 3.16b: Post sharp debridement by a podiatrist reveals the true extent of an underlying neuropathic ulcer

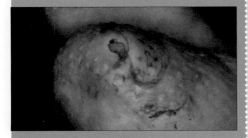

Figure 3.17: Apical ulcer which subsequently resulted in osteomyelitis

Superficial neuropathic ulcers require rapid treatment as they may soon penetrate to deeper structures such as bone.

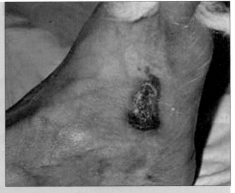

Figure 3.18: Ischaemic ulcer on the dorsal aspect of the foot due to poor footwear in a foot with peripheral arterial disease

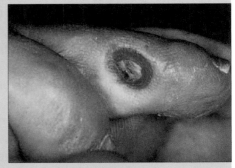

Figure 3.19: Inter-digital ischaemic ulceration on the lateral aspect of the toe as a result of tight shoes in a foot with peripheral arterial disease

Table 3.5: Vascular assessment

Palpation of foot pulses

Palpation of femoral or popliteal pulses if foot pulses are weak or absent

Use of a hand-held Doppler to locate foot pulses

Ankle brachial pressure index (ABPI) (*Box 3.11*)

Toe brachial pressure index (TBPI) (*Box 3.11*)

(Baker *et al*, 2005)

Patients presenting with lower limb ischaemia requiring revascularisation, for example, an ABPI of <0.5 without ulceration, or, <0.7 in the presence of ulceration, should be referred urgently to the vascular team.

Box 3.11: Vascular testing

ABPI

It has been suggested that 30% of patients with diabetes mellitus will have medial arterial calcification. Calcification of arteries can result in a falsely elevated ABPI ratio. Practitioners should be aware that calcification may be present even when a 'normal' ratio (0.98–1.2) is calculated.

(Marshall, 2004; Vowden, 1999)

TBPI

As calcification rarely extends to digital arteries, the TBPI has been suggested as a viable alternative to the ABPI when calcification is suspected.

(Marshall, 2004)

Infection

Infection in the neuroischaemic foot can rapidly give rise to cellulitis that often progresses to tissue necrosis (Edmonds, 2005; Hutchinson, 2000). Prompt diagnosis and treatment of infection yields the best clinical outcomes

(Giurini and Lyons, 2005). However, the signs and symptoms of infection are diminished in the neuroischaemic foot, making microbiological investigation to establish correct antibiotic therapy essential.

Prevention is the focus for those with no ulcerations. For those with ulcerations, prompt recognition and treatment is key (Giurini, 2005). Any potentially infected 'diabetic foot' must be taken seriously, and non-painful, deep sepsis suspected if there is evidence of sensory loss. Severe infection in the diabetic foot may need intravenous antibiotic therapy/surgical drainage and/or debridement. Infected neuroischaemic feet need vascular assessment and intervention where appropriate. It is equally important to maintain strict metabolic control and optimise cardiovascular function to improve the chances of wound healing (Edmonds, 2005).

Consideration should be given to eliminating nasal carriage of _staphylococci_ if recurrent superficial sepsis occurs in the presence of poor diabetic control.

Fungal infections, both of skin and nails, are common but usually not serious in the absence of immunosuppression. Treatment with topical antifungals may need to be combined with systemic therapy for successful eradication. Systemic antifungal therapy should be carefully considered as treatment needs to be prolonged and is potentially toxic, particularly in individuals with diabetes mellitus who often have co-morbidities.

Wound debridement

Wound debridement should include the removal of all dead and devitalised tissue to render infection less likely. Sharp debridement, by a skilled practitioner, provides a rapid means of removing necrotic tissue. Sharp debridement should only be attempted following thorough assessment, and caution should be exercised in the presence of ischaemia.

A recent systematic review investigated the effectiveness of debridement as a treatment for diabetic foot ulceration (_Box 3.12_).

Wound dressings

There is no single ideal wound dressing for the diabetic foot, and no evidence exists to suggest that any particular wound dressing is more effective for diabetic foot ulceration (American Diabetes Association, 2003). A plethora of wound dressings exist making dressing selection challenging for the practitioner. Thomas (1997) suggests that dressing selection should incorporate the following factors; wound type, wound location, wound characteristics, bacterial profile, product-related factors such as conformability, low adherence, antibacterial properties and patient-related factors such as compliance, the need to bathe, and activity levels.

Appropriate management of wound exudate is imperative to maintain a moist wound healing environment, however, the presence of excessive or uncontrolled exudate can result in peri-wound maceration. Maceration of the wound periphery can result in an increase in wound dimensions and wound excoriation (White and Cutting, 2004). Methods to avoid maceration are outlined in *Box 3.13*.

Box 3.12: Debridement

A recent systematic review (Smith, 2002) looked at the effectiveness of debridement as a treatment for diabetic foot ulcers in type 1 or type 2 patients. Hydrogel was slightly more effective than gauze or standard care in healing diabetic foot ulcers, and surgical debridement and larval therapy showed no significant benefit. However, of the five randomised controlled trials, sample sizes were predominantly small: <22 per group in three studies, and 70 per group in the other two studies.

Box 3.13: Avoidance of maceration

❖ Wound management products should be selected according to the volume of wound exudate present.
❖ Optimal wear time for wound dressings should not be exceeded.
❖ The amount of time advised between dressing changes should be estimated as objectively as possible.
❖ Infection should be managed appropriately.

(Stansfield, 2000; White and Cutting, 2004)

Peri-ulcer skin care

Approximately 30% of patients with diabetes mellitus will have disease-related dermatological problems. Therefore, effective wound management planning should include the protection of peri-ulcer tissues to prevent further complications arising. The following should be considered:

❖ Anhydrotic skin associated with autonomic neuropathy can give rise to fragile skin prone to fissuring, thus increasing the likelihood of opportunistic bacterial infection. Regular emollient use should be advocated.
❖ Callus may occur around the wound margins, particularly in the case of neuropathic ulceration. Callus should be debrided. Caution should be exercised in the presence of ischaemia.
❖ Contact dermatitis is a common reaction to topical products or other sensitisers. Many reactions are not apparent from history, and patch testing for sensitivity is recommended. Skin barrier products can be a useful adjunct to prevent skin irritation from adhesive dressings or tapes, particularly for individuals with atrophic or anhydrotic skin. Barrier products also have a role to play in the prevention of peri-ulcer maceration without hindering dressing adhesion.
❖ Circumferential tape or tight bandaging around the foot, particularly digits, can seriously compromise tissue perfusion and is contra-indicated in the diabetic foot (Stansfield, 2000).
❖ Varicose eczema should be treated by physical therapies intended to improve venous return and prevent peripheral oedema and tissue injury.

Off-loading the diabetic foot

In the presence of neuropathy, diabetic patients generally develop foot ulceration over sites of high pressure and shear on the plantar aspect of the foot, primarily related to normal walking (Armstrong _et al_, 2003). Superficial diabetic foot ulceration can rapidly become more extensive in the presence of repetitive stress during daily activities. The central goal of any management plan designed to facilitate healing should include strategies to reduce pressure. Removal of pressure, known as off-loading, can be achieved by a number of strategies, including avoidance of weight bearing, the use of irremovable and removable cast walkers, half shoes, orthotic devices, and therapeutic footwear.

The total contact cast (TCC) is considered to be the gold standard in redistribution of pressure over the plantar surface (Armstrong *et al*, 2005). However, in the presence of ischaemia and/or infection, the TCC may be contraindicated and an alternative strategy, such as a removable walker, allowing regular assessment of the wound, should be considered.

Therapeutic footwear is frequently prescribed as a management strategy in the primary and secondary prevention of diabetic foot ulceration, and as an adjunct to aid healing when ulceration is present. Maciejewski *et al* (2004) reviewed current evidence for the effectiveness of therapeutic shoes in preventing ulceration and found that several studies reported statistically significant protective benefits from therapeutic footwear.

Therapeutic footwear alone will not provide adequate pressure reduction and insole therapy is often indicated. A thorough assessment of the structure and mechanics of the foot should be undertaken by a podiatrist and/or orthotist prior to insole prescription.

Further reading and useful websites

National Institute for Clinical Excellence: http://www.nice.org.uk
Edmonds ME, Foster A, Sanders (2004) *A Practical Manual of Diabetic Footcare*. Blackwell Science, Oxford
Bowker JH, MA Pfiefer (2001) *Levin and O'Neal's The Diabetic Foot*. 6th edn. Mosby, USA
Boulton AJM, Connor H, Cavanagh PR *et al* (2000) *The Foot in Diabetes*. 3rd edn. John Wiley, Chichester

Conclusion

An estimated 1.3 million people in the United Kingdom have type 2 diabetes (NICE, 2004), consequently, the challenge of managing complications such as foot ulcers in diabetes care places a huge financial burden on the NHS. The patient with diabetes also suffers immeasureable costs in terms of their physical and psychosocial health.

The aims for healthcare practitioners to effectively manage the patient at risk of, or with foot ulceration, should be:

- seek to achieve the goals of the *NSF for Diabetes*
- embrace up-to-date evidence, eg. NICE guidance on the prevention and management of foot problems
- appreciate the complexities of managing diabetes from the patient's perspective through structured education models
- encourage communication between multi-agencies to realise optimal patient care through specialist diabetes foot clinics with fast track surgical referral mechanisms
- use knowledge and skills to be **ALERT** in early recognition of, and prompt treatment of, problems
- take a proactive role in order to **PREVENT** further damage to the vunerable diabetic foot.

In conclusion, evidence suggests that emphasis on early identification and prevention of diabetic foot ulcers, via early recognition of complications and identification of risk factors associated with diabetic foot ulceration, can minimise adverse outcomes and further complications.

References

Abouaesha F, Carine HM, Griffiths GD, Young RJ, Boulton AJM (2001) Plantar tissue thickness is related to peak plantar pressure in the high-risk diabetic foot. *Diabetes Care* **24**(7): 1270–4

American Diabetes Association (2003) Peripheral arterial disease in people with diabetes. *Diabetes Care* **26**(12): 3333–41

Armstrong DG *et al* (1998) Validation of a diabetic wound classification system. *Diabetes Care* **21**(5): 855–9

Armstrong DG, Lavery LA, Kimbriel HR *et al* (2003) Activity patterns of patients with diabetic foot ulceration. *Diabetes Care* **26**(9): 2595–7

Armstrong DG, Lavery LA, Wu S *et al* (2005) Evaluation of removable and irremovable cast walkers in the healing of diabetic foot wounds. *Diabetes Care* **28**(3): 551–4

Baker N, Murali-Krishnan S, Fowler D (2005) A user's guide to foot screening. Part 2: peripheral arterial disease. *The Diabetic Foot* **8**(2): 58–70

Boulton AJM, Connor H, Cavanagh PR *et al* (2000) The foot. In: *Diabetes*. 3rd edn. John Wiley, Chichester

Bowker JH, Pfiefer MA (2001) *Levin and O'Neal's The Diabetic Foot*. 6th edn. Mosby, USA

Buchman (2005) Biomechanical implications in offloading the diabetic foot (oral communication). The Biomechanics of Wounds and Wound Care conference, Oxford, UK

Currie CJ, Morgan CL, Peters JR (1998) The epidemiology and cost of inpatient care for peripheral vascular disease, infection, neuropathy, and ulceration in diabetes. *Diabetes Care* **21**(1): 42–8

Dealey C (2005) *The Care of Wounds. A Guide For Nurses*. 3rd edn. Blackwell Science, London

Department of Health (2005) *Structured Patient Education in Diabetes; Report from the patient education working group*. DoH, London

Department of Health (2001) *National service framework for diabetes: standards*. DoH, London

Diabetes Control and Complications Trial (DCCT) (1993) The effect of intensive treatment of diabetes on the development and progression of long term complications in insulin dependant diabetes mellitus. *N Eng J Med* **329**: 977–86

Edmonds M (2005) Infection in the neuroischaemic foot. *Int J Low Extrem Wounds* **4**: 145–53

Edmonds ME, Foster A, Sanders (2004) *A Practical Manual Of Diabetic Footcare*. Blackwell Science, Oxford

Edmonds M, Foster A (1999) *Managing the Diabetic Foot*. Blackwell Science, Oxford

Giurini J, Lyons T (2005) Diabetic foot complications: diagnosis and management. *Int J Low Extrem Wounds* **4**: 171–82

Hutchinson A *et al* (2000) *Clinical guidelines for type 2 diabetes: prevention and management of foot problems*. Royal College of General Practitioners, London

International Working Group on the Diabetic Foot (1999) International Consensus on the Diabetic Foot. Amsterdam, The Netherlands

Kumar S, Ashe HA, Parnell LN *et al* (1994) The prevalence of foot ulceration and its correlates in Type 2 diabetic patients: a population based study. *Diabetic Med* **11**: 480–4

Maciejewski ML, Reiber GE, Smith DG *et al* (2004) Effectiveness of diabetic therapeutic footwear in preventing reulceration. *Diabetes Care* **27**(7) 1774–82

Marshall C (2004) The ankle: brachial pressure index. A critical appraisal. *Br J Podiatry* **7**(4): 93–5

Murray HJ, Young MJ, Hollis S *et al* (1996) The association between callus formation, high pressures and neuropathy in diabetic foot ulceration. *Diabetes Med* **13**: 979–82

National Institute for Clinical Excellence (2004) Clinical guidelines for Type 2 diabetes: Prevention and management of foot problems, clinical guideline 10. NICE, London

Neil HAW, Thompson AV, Thorogood M (1989) Diabetes in the elderly: The Oxford Community Diabetes Study. *Diabetic Med* **6**: 608–13

Plank J, Haas W, Rakovac I *et al* (2003) Evaluation of the impact of chiropodist care in the secondary prevention of foot ulcerations in diabetic subjects. *Diabetes Care* **26**(6): 1691–5

Ronnemaa T, Hamalainen H, Toikka T *et al* (1997) Evaluation of the impact of podiatrist care in the primary prevention of foot problems in diabetic subjects. *Diabetes Care* **20**: 1833–7

Smith J (2002) *Debridement of diabetic foot ulcers* (Cochrane review). Citation: Smith J. Debridement of diabetic foot ulcers. The Cochrane Database of Systematic Reviews 2002, Issue 4. Art. No: CD003556. DOI: 10.1002/14651858.CD003556

Stansfield G (2000) Managing wound exudate in the diabetic foot ulcer. *The Diabetic Foot* **3**(3): 93–7

The Cochrane Database of Systematic Reviews 2005 Issue 3. Copyright © 2005 The Cochrane Collaboration. Published by John Wiley and Sons, Ltd, Chichester

Thomas S (1997) A Structured Approach to the selection of Dressings. World Wide Wounds. Available online at: http://www.worldwidewounds.com/1997/july/Thomas-Guide/Dress-Select.html (accessed 11/09/05)

UK Prospective Diabetes Study (1998) Intensive blood-glucose control with sulphonylureas or insulin compared with conventional treatment and risk of complications in patients with type 2 diabetes. (UKPDS 33) *Lancet* **352**(9131): 837–53

Vowden P (1999) Doppler ultrasound in the management of the diabetic foot. *Diabetic Foot J* supplement **2**(1): 16–7

Walters DA, Gatling W, Mullee MA, Hill RD (1992) The distribution and severity of diabetic foot disease: a community based study with comparison to a non-diabetic group. *Diabetic Med* **9**: 354–58

White RJ, Cutting KC (2004). Maceration of the skin and wound bed by indication. In: White R, ed. *Trends in Wound Care*, volume III. Quay Books, MA Healthcare Limited, London

Young M *et al* (1992) The effect of callus removal on dynamic foot pressures in diabetic patients. *Diabetes Med* **9**: 55–7

Chapter 4

Skin trauma

Clare Morris

Introduction

The promotion and maintenance of skin integrity is one of the most common challenges for nurses in every sphere of practice (Voegeli, 2005). The maintenance of healthy skin depends on factors such as moisture, nutritional status of the patient and mechanical forces (Hampton, 2004).

As skin ages, the dermis thins by approximately 20% due to a reduction in collagen and elastin. This is especially after the age of seventy years and is consistently thinner in women than in men (Desai, 1997). The blood supply also decreases, leading to poorer regulation of the skin's surface temperature and increased pallor.

Skin trauma wounds can range from scratches or minor cuts to extensive burns and crush injuries (Benbow, 2005). This chapter will focus on the management of the minor traumatic wounds as outlined in *Table 4.1*.

Accurate assessment of the minor traumatic wound is important to confirm the full extent or minor nature of the injury, and to rule out any fractures, foreign bodies or nerve injury. Although the wound may be classed as 'minor', the patient may still feel pain and anxiety, therefore, reassurance and explanation of treatment are important (Ballard and Baxter, 2000).

Table 4.1: Minor traumatic wounds
❖ Skin tears
❖ Lacerations
❖ Minor burns/scalds
❖ Contusions or bruises
❖ Haematomas
❖ Abrasions
❖ Bites
❖ Pruritus and scratching

There are three key elements or general principles to consider when assessing a minor injury:

1. Accurate description of the wound and establish if the wound is contaminated or clean.
2. Documentation of the mechanism or nature and cause of the injury, status of tetanus immunisation, current medication and known allergies.
3. First aid measures for haemostasis, cleansing of the wound and the surrounding skin ensuring identification and removal of foreign bodies, temporary closure of the wound by re-opposing skin edges where possible/appropriate.

Other important considerations are:

- ensuring the wound dressing is atraumatic to the wound bed
- adequate pain relief by using appropriate dressing and simple analgesia
- providing comfort and maintaining normal function
- giving information on the healing process, signs and symptoms of wound infection/complications and clinic or community follow-up (Ballard and Baxter, 2000; Benbow, 2005).

Skin tears

Skin tears are a common problem in the elderly because the skin atrophies and becomes thin and fragile (Meuleneire, 2002). They commonly occur on the shinbone and on the arm. Skin tears are caused by friction, or, a combination of shearing and friction forces. Skin tears can be described as partial- or full-thickness wounds (Payne and Martin, 1993). Partial-thickness means superficial damage of the epidermis; full-thickness involves deeper tissues of the dermis and small blood vessels.

Payne and Martin (1993) developed a classification system to help formulate guidelines for practice.

❖ Category 1 — skin tears with no loss of tissue:

- linear type: epidermis and dermis are pulled in one layer from the supporting structures

- flap type: epidermis and dermis are separated, but the epidermal flap covers the dermis to within 1mm of the wound margin.

❖ Category 2 — this comprises two types:

- scant loss of tissue (up to 25%)
- moderate to large loss of tissue (25% or more of the flap has disappeared during trauma).

❖ Category 3 — skin tears that involve the entire loss of tissue; it can be caused by the initial trauma, or the flap becoming necrotic. Traditional methods of management include removal of the skin flap immediately after the trauma, suturing, or the use of Steri-Strip™ skin closures. Due to the nature of fragile skin combined with inflammatory action, extra care should be taken to prevent further damage and delayed wound healing.

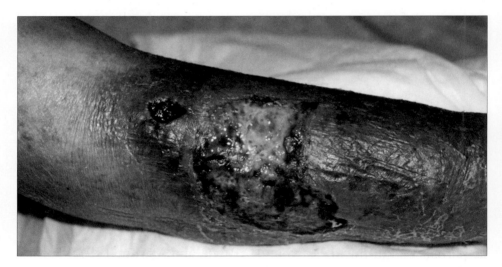

Figure 4.1: Category 3 skin tear with a complete loss of tissue

The aim of wound management in these wounds is to stop bleeding, prevent infection, recover skin integrity, minimise pain and promote patient comfort (Payne and Martin, 1993). Suitable wound dressings include the following:

- soft silicone membranes/membranes
- soft silicone foam/foam

- hydrogels/sheet hydrogels for dry necrotic tissue
- Hydrofiber®/alginates for high levels of exudate.

Some deep skin tears with large tissue loss may require skin grafting.

Lacerations

Lacerations are breaches or splits in the skin caused by a blunt instrument or force, eg. the result of a fall, crushing injury or blow with a blunt instrument over a bony prominence (Benbow, 2005).

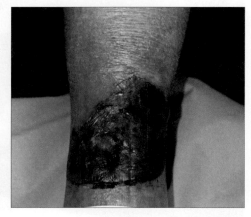

Pre-tibial lacerations are a common injury occurring most often in older women (Bradley, 2001). They affect the skin overlying the anterior aspect of the tibial bone (Dearden *et al*, 2001), especially the distal third of the pre-tibial region (Bradley, 2001).

Figure 4.2: Pre-tibial laceration including subcutaneous tissue

They can range from a neat linear shape with minimal tissue loss, to a tearing type of cut with a jagged wound edge and devitalised tissue (Dearden *et al*, 2001). They may be superficial with skin loss only, or may extend to full thickness, including subcutaneous tissue.

Classically, the wound contains a V-shaped flap of tissue that is attached on one side only. A bluish tinge to the flap edge usually indicates that its blood supply has been compromised (Dearden *et al*, 2001).

The aim of wound management is to reunite the opposing wound edges (Young, 1997). Traditionally, practitioners have treated pre-tibial lacerations conservatively by cleansing, debridement and approximating the wound edges, however, this may be associated with delayed healing rates and protracted use of wound dressings (Bradley, 2001).

Bradley (2003) discusses the role of graduated compression therapy in the management of pre-tibial lacerations. It is essential that prior to the decision to use graduated compression therapy, a full medical and vascular assessment is made, including ankle brachial pressure index

(ABPI) measurements to determine the patient's arterial status. Graduated compression increases venous return, and reduces hydrostatic pressure and oedema. The use of graduated compression therapy will depend on the vascular status of the limb and the condition of the patient's skin, as high compression can damage fragile skin (Bradley, 2001).

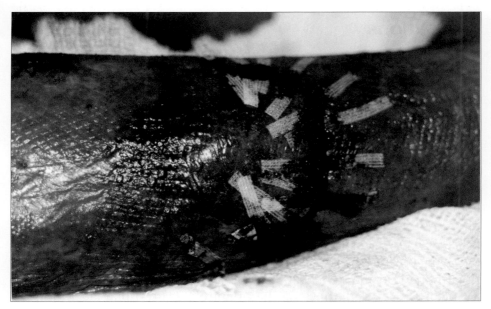

Figure 4.3: Pre-tibial laceration secured with Steri-Strip™ skin closures, holding the v-shaped flap of skin in place

Minor burns and scalds

There are various definitions of what constitutes a minor burn or scald injury. One commonly used classification for minor burns is a partial-thickness burn, involving less than 5% body surface area in an adult (Gower, 1996 in Fowler, 1999).

The National Burn Injury Referral Guidelines (2001) give a comprehensive guide on when a burn is likely to be complex. Accurate assessment of burn-injured patients is required to differentiate between complex and non-complex burns (Lloyd-Jones, 2001).

The depth of tissue penetrated by the burn determines the classification. The various grades are defined as:

- superficial
- superficial partial-thickness
- deep partial-thickness (deep dermal)
- full-thickness (Fowler, 1999).

In a superficial burn involving the epidermis, the skin is dry, intact, red, very painful and blanches under pressure. There is minimal tissue damage, and a blister may form up to forty-eight hours after the initial injury. Healing is usually rapid and uncomplicated, occurring within three to seven days with minimal treatment.

Superficial partial-thickness burns involve the epidermis and superficial dermis. They blister immediately, are red in areas and are moist and exuding. They have a brisk capillary refill, which blanches under pressure, and are very painful being especially sensitive to the air and temperature. They usually heal within ten to twenty-one days if no infection is present (Fowler, 1999).

The range of treatments for burns varies enormously according to the depth, severity and extent of the injury (Benbow, 2005). The aim of wound care in burns is to:

- maintain a clean, moist environment
- promote patient comfort
- offer protection from infection or other trauma
- facilitate optimal activity and function (Fowler, 1999).

The initial first aid measure is to apply cool water for ten to twenty minutes, with the exception of electrical injuries, facial burns and certain chemical agents.

Dressings commonly used in superficial and partial-thickness burns are:

- hydrocolloids/thin hydrocolloids
- hydrogels/sheet hydrogels
- silicone membranes/silicone foam
- foams
- alginates/Hydrofiber® for high exudate.

Contusions or bruises

Bruises or contusions occur as a result of the rupture of subcutaneous or deeper blood vessels following an impact (Benbow, 2005). They are usually the result of a direct blow and unlike abrasions, which occur at the point of impact, bruises may occur at sites away from the injured part of the body (Evans and Jones, 1996).

Bleeding and oedema from increased capillary permeability cause pain and swelling of the injured area. If the bruise is small, no treatment is required. Larger bruises may lead to a haematoma.

Haematomas

Haematomas are localised collections of extravasated blood which are either totally, or relatively, confined within a tissue space (Evans and Jones, 1996).

Treatment is mainly the prevention of further bleeding and evacuation or promotion of absorption of the blood.

Complications of haematoma include:

* infection
* skin necrosis
* compartment syndrome
* hypovolaemia/blood loss.

Initial treatment is to elevate the area and the application of ice. Pressure dressings may also be useful. Large haematomas that are causing pressure need to be aspirated or surgically evacuated.

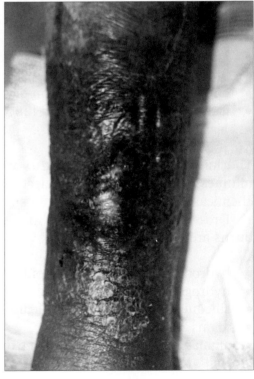

Figure 4.4: Haematoma within the tissue space

Absorption of blood may be accelerated by local application of heat and ultrasound, although the evidence is not conclusive.

When a haematoma occurs within a muscle, gentle mobilisation within the limits of pain may aid resorption (Evans and Jones, 1996).

Wound dressings are used to maintain a warm, moist environment, and to facilitate debridement or evacuation of blood. They include the amorphous hydrogels or sheet hydrogels, Hydrofiber® and alginates.

Abrasions

These wounds are shear and friction injuries that result in a scraping or rubbing away of the epidermis or dermis (Flynn, 1994). They are superficial wounds that can be extremely painful due to exposed nerve endings (Young, 1997).

Abrasions can vary in depth depending on the extent of epidermal and dermal loss. The majority of these injuries tend to be superficial but, occasionally, the fascia and bone may also be involved (Evans and Jones, 1996).

Abrasions often contain dirt and other foreign material. Meticulous attention must always be paid to cleansing and to debridement as, once healing has occurred, it is almost impossible to remove any debris trapped in the dermis, and unsightly 'tattooing' results (Evans and Jones, 1996).

Treatment of abrasions should include the following:

- analgesia, cleansing and debridement
- occlusive dressing to encourage rapid healing, reduce pain and reduce the risk of infection, eg. hydrocolloid or semi-permeable film
- tetanus prophylaxis.

Bites

This section shall discuss human and dog bites as they make up the largest proportion of all bites. A review of other animal bites including cats, rats, squirrels, snakes and bats can be found in Higgins _et al_ (1997).

A bite wound can range from a superficial scratch to a major tear (Dearden *et al*, 2001). All bites have the potential to introduce bacteria deep into the soft tissues where, after a short incubation period, they may proliferate and spread. Human bites are potentially the most infective bite (Bradley and Collier, 1994).

Human bite wounds are the second most frequently reported bite and constitute 18% of all bites (Higgins *et al*, 1997). They are second to dog bites. Petersen and Ryan (1996) report that 30% of all human bites become infected. The commonest aerobes associated with human bites are *Staphylococcus aureus* and *streptococci*. Other pathogens such as human immunodeficiency virus (HIV), hepatitis B and C, syphilis, tuberculosis and tetanus can all be transmitted by human bites (Higgins *et al*, 1997).

Dog bites account for 74% of bite wounds and occur most often in children (*Figure 4.5*) (Higgins *et al*, 1997). Dog bites carry a moderate risk of becoming infected.

The management of patients with bite wounds includes the following:

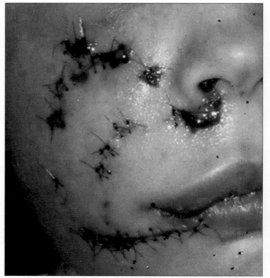

Figure 4.5: A facial dog bite that has been sutured

* Thorough history and examination:
  * identification of animal species
  * time elapsed since injury
  * skin condition
  * wound depth
  * degree of crush injury
  * damage to nerves, tendons, bones and joints
  * X-ray if suspect fractures or foreign bodies
  * past medical history and risk factors
  * tetanus status.

* Treatment, to include:
  * cleansing
  * debridement
  * primary or delayed primary closure

- antibiotics if indicated
- admission if indicated
- tetanus prophylaxis.

Not all wounds require antibiotics. Risk factors should be identified from history and examination (Higgins _et al_, 1997).

Whenever possible, wounds should be allowed to heal by secondary intention and should not be sutured. The exception is facial wounds as they have an excellent blood supply and low incidence of infection.

Bite wounds should be assessed on a daily basis due to the high risk of spreading infection (Dearden _et al_, 2001).

Pruritus and scratching

Itching and dryness of the skin are two of the most commonly encountered problems affecting elderly patients (Graham-Brown and Monk, 1988). Pruritus or itching may arise from many different sources. Examples of systemic disorders associated with generalised pruritus in the elderly are:

- chronic renal failure — possibly due to urea
- cholestatic liver disease — due to bile salts and signals bilary obstruction
- thyroid disease — found in hyper and hypothyroidism
- iron deficiency
- malignant disease — especially in Hodgkin's disease.

It is important that screening tests are performed to try and ensure that none of these are missed.

Pruritus can lead to scratching which can cause trauma to the skin.

Allergies to wound care products can lead to irritant

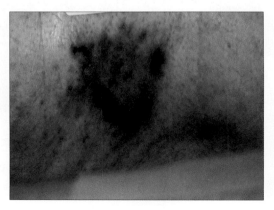

Figure 4.6: A Scratch wound with superficial skin loss

83

and inflammatory reactions, resulting in allergic contact dermatitis or irritant dermatitis (Young, 2000). The treatment for allergic contact dermatitis starts with patch testing to identify a reaction on the skin. The treatment for irritant dermatitis relies upon the identification of the irritant substance and its subsequent avoidance (Young, 2000).

Scratching of dry, irritated skin can lead to tissue breakdown and occurrence of ulceration (Newton and Cameron, 2003), or, the extension of existing ulcerated areas (Cameron and Powell, 1992).

Topical steroids can be used to ease the discomfort. Long-term, emollients can help maintain skin hydration and barrier function (Voegeli, 2005).

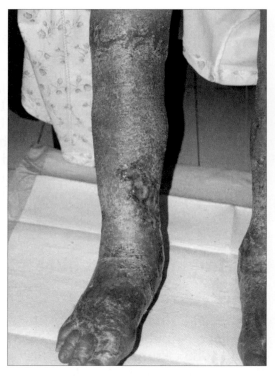

Figure 4.7: Dry, itchy skin surrounding a leg ulcer

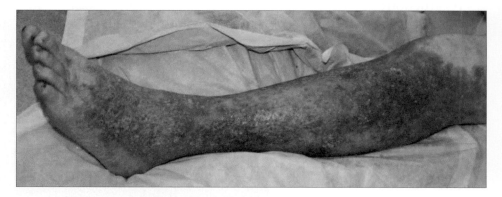

Figure 4.8: Contact dermatitis due to the components of a bandage

The skin is covered with microorganisms (skin flora), the most common inhabitant being bacteria. Bacteria are generally part of the natural balance and are, on the whole, harmless. However, once there is a break in the skin, for example from scratching dry varicose eczema, the bacteria can enter and become established in the tissue causing cellulitis (inflammation of subcutaneous tissue) (Hampton and Collins, 2003; Hampton, 2004).

References

Ballard K, Baxter H (2000) *Essential wound healing part 7: managing acute wounds.* EMAP Healthcare, London, UK

Benbow M (2005) *Evidence-based Wound Management.* Whurr Publications, London

Bradley D, Collier M (1994) Principles of trauma and the treatment of traumatic wounds. Wound Care Society Education Leaflet 2(3.

Bradley L (2001) Pretibial lacerations in older patients: the treatment options. *J Wound Care* **10**(1): 521–3

Bradley L (2003) Practical issues in the management of superficial pre-tibial skin tears in the older person. *Nurse 2 Nurse* **3**(3): 42–4

Cameron J, Powell S (1992) Contact dermatitis: its importance in leg ulcer patients. *Wound Management* **2**(3): 12–13

Dearden C, Donnell J, Donnelly J, Dunlop M (2001) Traumatic wounds: local wound management. *Nurs Times* **97**(35): 55–7

Desai H (1997) Ageing and wounds part 2: healing in old age. *J Wound Care* **6**(5): 237–9

Evans RC, Jones NL (1996) The management of abrasions and bruises. *J Wound Care* **5**(10): 465–8

Flynn MB (1994) Wound management of the traumatically injured patient. *Crit Care Nurs Clin N Am* **6**(3): 491–9

Fowler A (1999) Burns. In: Miller M, Glover D, eds. *Wound Management Theory and Practice.* EMAP Healthcare, London, UK.

Gower J (1996) *Report of the burns working group.* North and South Thames NHS region, London

Graham-Brown RAC, Monk BE (1988) Pruritus and xerosis. In: Monk BE, Graham-Brown RAC, Sarkany I, eds. *Skin Disorders in the Elderly.* Blackwell Scientific Publications, Oxford

Hampton S (2004) The nursing care of common raw and bleeding skin conditions. *Br J Nurs* **13**(10): 618–20

Hampton S, Collins F (2003) *Tissue Viability*. Whurr Publications, London

Higgins MAG, Evans RC, Evans RJ (1997) Managing animal and bite wounds. *J Wound Care* **6**(8): 377–80

Lloyd-Jones M (2001) Burns. *Practice Nurse* **22**(6) 41–4

Meuleneire F (2002) Using a soft silicone coated-net dressing to manage skin tears. *J Wound Care* **11**(10): 365–9

National Burn Care Review Committee Report (2001) *Standards and Strategy for Burn Care*. British Association of Plastic Surgeons, London

Newton H, Cameron J (2003) *Skin Care in Wound Management*. Medical Communications UK Ltd, Holsworthy

Payne RL, Martin ML (1993) Defining and classifying skin tears: need for a common language. *Ostomy Wound Management* **93**(3): 16–26

Petersen G, Ryan T (1996) Animal and human bites. *Wound Management* **2**: 9

Voegeli D (2005) Skin hygiene practices, emollient therapy and skin vulnerability. *Nurs Times supplement* **101**(4): 57–9

Young T (1997) Wound care in the accident and emergency department. *Br J Nurs* **6**(7): 395–01

Young T (2000) Assessing possible allergies to wound care products. *Community Nurse* **6**(8): 65–6

CHAPTER 5

SKIN MACERATION: ASSESSMENT, PREVENTION AND TREATMENT

Sylvie Hampton and Jackie Stephen-Haynes

Introduction

The human skin is well suited to serve as a barrier to our environment (*Chapter 1*). It is, however, compromised when challenged with wounding and chemical effects, such as interaction with detergents, solvents, and, excess water. This latter situation occurs when wound exudate, urine, or faeces come into contact with the skin for prolonged periods. Over-hydration of the epidermis will lead to softening of the tissues or 'maceration' (Scanlon and Stubbs, 2004). Wound exudate, particularly from chronic wounds, is often responsible for causing maceration of the surrounding skin. This chapter will review the reasons for that common problem.

Fluid from acute wounds may have a beneficial effect on wound healing, as it is rich with growth factors and, the necessary acute inflammation with all the components, to promote healing. However, chronic wounds are in a state of chronic inflammation and all the elements of normal wound healing are dysfunctional. The exudate of chronic wounds can have a negative effect (Vowden and Vowden, 2004), and this will be examined later in this chapter.

The acceptable level of fluid in a wound

A degree of moisture is essential for moist wound healing (Winter, 1963), however, the correct moisture balance is, as yet, difficult to define and no one has been able to qualify an acceptable level. Collier (2003) has attempted to clarify it by describing, 'an optimal moist environment — not too wet, not too dry — reducing the risk of complications to the surrounding skin'. This suggests that wounds that are too dry will not heal optimally, and wounds that are too wet will deteriorate (Bishop *et al*, 2003). Avoidance of these extremes is clearly the strategy, which is best achieved by the routine assessment of:

- skin
- wound
- incontinence
- peri-wound skin
- exudate.

Large volumes of exudate can, if inappropriately managed, lead to saturation of the wound bed and peri-wound area, resulting in their maceration (Cutting, 1999; White and Cutting, 2003). Related to this is excoriation, which is inflammation of the epidermis caused by chemical disruption of the stratum corneum due to an irritant, such as a chemical, bacteria or body fluids (Scanlon, 2004).

Causes of maceration

There is a tendency to think of maceration as an exclusively wound-related phenomenon. This is not strictly accurate, as maceration can involve skin that is remote from exuding wounds: for example, areas exposed to urine or sweaty, moist areas such as the feet and between skin folds. Other causes of maceration include:

1. Overhydration of the epidermis.
2. Use of inappropriate dressings or incorrect wear time.
3. Failure to protect the skin.
4. Destruction of the tissues through the effects of proteolytic enzymes in chronic wound exudate.

The theory of moist wound healing (Winter, 1963) espoused the benefits of moisture to achieve healing within an acute wound. Wound exudate originates from the blood circulation. Chronic wounds may lead to malfunctioning capillaries leaking serous fluid. This is caused by stimulation from inflammatory mediators, bacterial toxins and, in the case of venous leg ulcers, defective lymphatic drainage associated with vascular disease. The most significant complication caused by inadequate exudate control is maceration. This has been defined as 'the softening of tissue that has remained moist or wet for a long period' (Collins _et al_, 2002). It has been suggested that this is an under-recognised problem that causes delayed healing (White and Cutting, 2003). Maceration appears as a white and soggy tissue (_Figure 5.1_), which may lead to the break-down of the peri-wound area and enlargement of the wound (Cutting and White, 2004). Dressing leakage, wound pain, and prolonged healing time, can also lead to deterioration in quality of life for the patient (Vowden and Vowden, 2004).

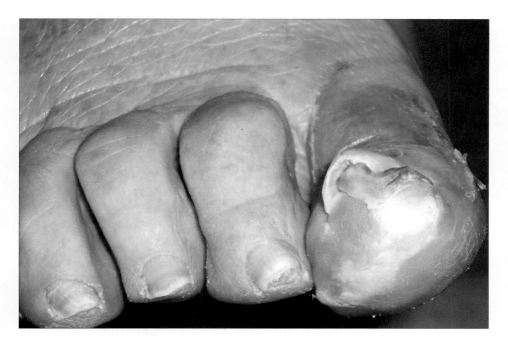

Figure 5.1: Maceration in the great toe

One of the causes of increased wound exudate is infection and/or critical colonisation (White _et al_, 2001). This can present significant management challenges. Specific bacteria present in the wound are responsible for an increase in protease enzymes (eg. elastases and other matrix metalloproteinases [MMPs]) which can, if in contact with the surrounding skin, cause excoriation and maceration (Cameron and Powell, 1992).

Role and pathology of proteolytic enzymes

Human skin is covered with commensal microorganisms (skin flora), the most common inhabitants being bacteria. There is a fine balance between environmental microorganisms and skin flora. This balance is maintained in an equilibrium, determined by conditions such as skin moisture and pH balance (Thompson, 1998), until there is a break in the protective layer which is the skin (Heggers, 1998). The exposed subcutaneous tissues provide a favourable substratum for a wide variety of mircoorganisms to contaminate and colonise (Bowler *et al*, 2001). Therefore, these bacteria are a part of the natural balance and are, on the whole, harmless, although, within a wound, the organisms can multiply and become pathogenic.

The inevitable colonisation of wounds is generally due to a mixture of species (Bowler *et al*, 2001) with aerobic pathogens, such as *Staphylococcus aureus* and *Pseudomonas aeruginosa* being cited as the most common, problematic, inhabitants (reviewed by Bowler *et al*, 2001). These organisms are 'water-loving', reflecting the wet environment in the wound with 88% of patients with uninfected leg ulcers being colonised with *Staphylococcus aureus* (Hansson *et al*, 1995). Additionally, many compromised wounds are contaminated with bacteria that also have the ability to add to the pool of proteases in the wound. For instance, *Pseudomonas aeruginosa*, which is found in 20%–30% of venous leg ulcers, can secrete both elastases and other proteases which might disrupt healing (Schmidtchen *et al*, 2001) (*Figure 5.2*).

Danielsen *et al* (1997) suggest that extra-cellular toxins produced by bacteria might also interfere with the healing process, with the responsible bacterial enzymes and metalloproteinase degrading fibrin and wound growth factors. At the same time, bacterial by-products (proteolytic enzymes and dead white cells) increase the viscosity of exudate and create a characteristic odour that can cause distress for both patient and carer (Bowler and Davies, 1999).

A pathological feature associated with some leg ulcers is the abnormally high level of proteolytic activity in the wound fluid, compared to the activity in wound fluid of normally healing wounds (Hoffman and Eagle, 1999). Fluid from chronic wounds contains high concentrations of protease enzymes, which may cause excessive degradation of extracellular matrix components, growth factors and growth factor receptors, thus contributing to the refractory nature of chronic wounds.

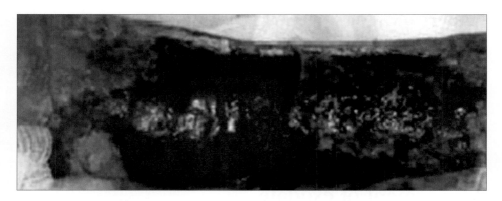

Figure 5.2: Tissues destroyed by *Pseudomonas*

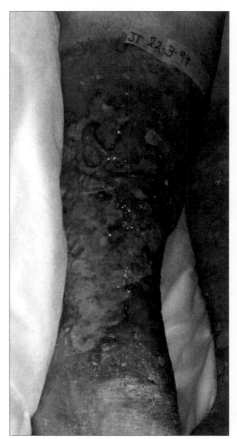

Proteolytic enzymes catalyse the breakdown of protein and are involved in the remodelling phase of wound healing. It is well-documented that chronic wounds exhibit elevated protease levels compared to healing acute wounds (Agren, 1994). Protease activity is regulated, in part, by naturally occurring inhibitors known as tissue inhibitors of metalloproteases (TIMPs), and the levels of these are reduced in chronic wound exudate (Brew *et al*, 2000).

Proteolytic enzymes from exudate can actually delay wound healing by reducing fibrolynitic activity (Phillips *et al*, 1998) and exacerbate skin damage through irritation (Cameron and Powell, 1996). This kind of tissue disruption by enzymes can be seen in *Figures 5.1* and *5.2*. Chronic wound exudate contains bacteria and protease enzymes and should be kept away from peri-wound skin as it is a wounding agent in its own right (Wysocki *et al*, 1993; Trengove *et al*, 1996).

A wound that has become 'chronic' is susceptible to bacterial

Figure 5.3: The straight demarcation line indicates the level of the dressing and the level that the wound fluid reaches in destruction of the tissue

invasion because of the warm, moist, protein-rich environment provided through wound exudate. Contamination or colonisation, particularly through skin flora, is a certain consequence (Leaper, 1994). Nevertheless, the organisms will often live within the wound and not clinically infect the host tissues, but there is the potential that these bacteria-laden fluids will spill over onto the skin and cause damage in the form of maceration and tissue destruction (*Figures 5.3* and *5.4*).

Assessment of exudate

The most desirable preventative strategy is to avoid maceration. However, determining the level of exudate has defied easy measurement. A brief review of articles over the last ten years has highlighted a number of approaches to assessment of exudate.

Wound exudate is generally regarded as the fluid that originates from incision or exposed tissue. Mulder (1994) suggested that exudate volume be determined by dressing usage. Indeed, the frequency of dressing changes is dictated by the requirements of the wound, a good indication to the amount or level of exudate. Consider a wound that requires a daily dressing change, or one where the dressing can be left in place for up to seven days. Consider also, the types of dressing that would be used in each instance. These actions do not adequately measure or describe the exudate, but they allow the subjective estimation of the level of fluid loss.

Young (1997) observed that one way of measuring exudate was to consider the colour, amount, and consistency, but that volume estimation was too subjective. Thomas (1997) and, more latterly Cutting (2004), observed the use of subjective measures using terms such as low, medium, high or +, ++, +++. Each of these systems can mean different things to each individual assessor.

Exudate varies in its consistency, being usually serous (watery, serum-like), although occasionally it is sero-sanguinous (with blood), or purulent (thick, opaque, malodorous) (exudate assessment and composition has been reviewed by Cutting, 2004). Assessment of exudate according to volume and viscosity (consistency) is described in the Wound Exudate Continuum (White and Gray, 2005), and is central to the system of Applied Wound Management (Gray *et al*, 2005). Vowden and Vowden (2004) suggest that assessment and management of exudate should include six 'C' factors (*Table 5.1*).

Table 5.1: The six 'Cs' (Vowden and Vowden, 2004)

Cause	Control	Components	Containment	Correction	Complications
Systemic local wound related.	Whether effective systemic or local control is possible.	Bacterial load. Necrotic tissue. Chemical composition, pH. Viscosity and volume.	Dressing seal at the wound surface; within the dressing — away from the wound and skin.	Control bacterial load (bioburden). Debridement. Exudate modification.	Maceration: skin protection. Protein loss. Pain. Odour.

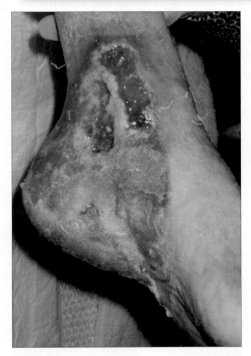

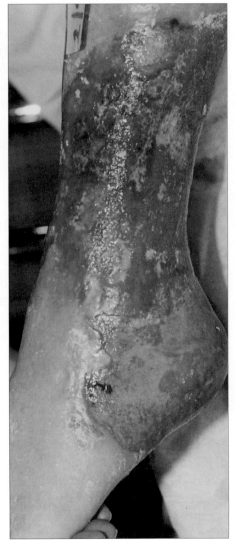

Figure 5.4: Exudate has spilled over onto the good skin. The direction of the fluid is according to gravity (dependent leakage)

Figure 5.5: Exudate has caused maceration. Note the straight demarcation lines that suggest this is excoriation and not infection

The components of *Table 5.1* suggest that addressing the cause, controlling or containing the exudate, and preventing complications will preserve skin integrity.

Preserving skin integrity

Wound exudate in the optimal volume and constituency is a useful component of the healing process, as it provides the 'moist' component in moist wound healing. Excessive wound exudate, or bodily fluids, such as urine or sweat, can cause skin maceration (around a wound or between excess skin folds, in the groin, etc) which may delay healing or lead to other complications and practitioners are advised to try to avoid it (Cutting and White, 2002; White and Cutting, 2003).

To avoid maceration and optimise healing:

- exudate levels should be regularly assessed
- suitable dressings chosen
- realistic wear times estimated for each wound at every dressing change (Cutting and White, 2002).

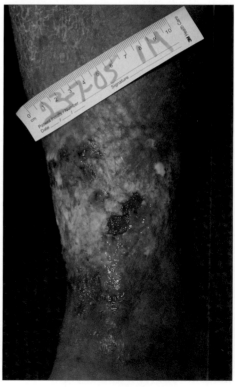

The skin acts as a passive barrier to many chemicals and infective agents (*Chapter 1*) until the epidermis is breached. When in the bath for a prolonged period of time, our skin becomes wrinkled and softened. This same process occurs around wound margins when exudate is constantly present. This softening of the tissues, along with constant irritation from proteolytic enzymes, can lead to a breach in the epidermis. Preserving skin integrity is one of the primary functions of the nurse: a complex and difficult task,

Figure 5.6: Maceration. *Pseudomonas* was present in this wound

especially in the case of chronic wounds when exudate can be a constant problem (Hampton, 2004).

Nevertheless, care of the peri-wound area relies largely on four key elements:

1. Reduction and/or control of wound exudate.
2. Reduction of wound bacteria if critically colonised or infected.
3. Protection of the skin.
4. Treatment of wet eczema.

Exudate management

The dressing of an exuding wound demands careful selection of appropriate dressing(s). This can be problematic as dressings are often only available in a narrow range of sizes and shapes. The mismatch that can occur between the size and shape of a wound and the available dressings can cause leakage, leading to maceration (Cowley *et al*, 2004). Therefore, exudate management depends critically on dressing selection, fit and optimum absorption and venting of excess fluid (Grocott, 1998). Some dressings will absorb fluid and will 'lock' it away, while others will reduce horizontal wicking of fluid and retain the exudate over the wound without touching the intact skin (Vowden and Vowden, 2004).

Reduction of exudate relies on absorption capabilities of the dressing, compression therapy in venous ulceration, and reduction of bacteria. The latter will reduce production of exogenous proteolytic enzymes.

Dressing selection

Management of maceration can be achieved through the use of appropriate, absorbent dressings, combined with a realistic wear time — extending wear time for convenience can lead to problems. Appropriate wear time, with the concomitant use of skin protectants is helpful (Williams, 2001; Neander and Hesse, 2003; Baatenberg de Jong and Admiraal, 2004; Graham *et al*, 2004).

Reduction of proteolytic enzymes

As proteolytic enzymes can be associated with maceration, and exogenous enzymes are of bacterial origin, it would be wise to consider a reduction of bacterial bioburden in a wound to reduce the exudate production (White *et al*, 2001). This reduction can be achieved through a variety of interventions, such as the use of antibacterial dressings. There are many types of antibacterial dressings on the market, all of which have a role to play in reducing microorganisms in a wound. It is important to be aware that all chronic wounds are colonised by bacteria, and that reduction of bioburden is not always necessary. The use of topical antimicrobials must be justified in each instance. Proteolytic enzymes are also of endogenous (neutrophil) origin; where these are suspected of compromising healing, alternative interventions exist.

Protection of the skin

Absorbent dressings can leak and are often changed only after leakage has occurred. As a result, the surrounding skin is exposed to wound exudate on a frequent or prolonged basis (Goldberg *et al*, 2000; Newman *et al*, 2001). Therefore, it is wise to change the dressing before the wound becomes saturated. This is often difficult to achieve, particularly when community nurses have set days to visit the patient. The only option open to this problem is to select realistic wear times.

Traditionally, both zinc oxide and petrolatum ointments have been routinely used to protect the peri-wound area. This approach is effective but can be problematic. These products can interfere with dressing function, such as absorption and adhesion, and are also messy to use and difficult to remove (Sibbald and Cameron, 2001; Cameron *et al*, 2005), and this takes up considerable nursing time (Cameron *et al*, 2005).

With the advent of liquid film-forming technologies, new skin barrier products have been developed for this protective need (Rolstad and Harris, 1997). These products form a continuous uniform barrier film on the skin surface. One of these newer technologies (Cavilon™ No Sting Barrier Film) provides a flexible, durable, breathable, moisture-repellent film on the skin (Rolstad and Harris, 1997; Cameron *et al*, 2005). Cavilon™ is also available in the form of a barrier cream (Cavilon™ Durable Barrier Cream), a water-in-oil emulsion that does not interfere with the function or adhesion of dressings (Williams, 2001). Both zinc and Cavilon™ Durable

Barrier Cream are effective barrier preparations, although Cavilon™ Cream is easy to apply and transparent.

There are other preparations that successfully protect the skin, although care must be taken to ensure that the function and adhesion of the dressing is not compromised by the type that is used. The difference in _Figures 5.2_ and _5.7_ demonstrates how the skin can be protected against damaging fluid and enzymes.

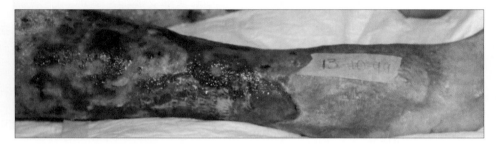

Figure 5.7: This is the same example as _Figure 5.2_. Protecting the skin has allowed healing to occur. Again, note the straightforward demarcation lines

Treatment of wet eczema

The use of topical corticosteroids is controversial but, for leg ulcers, they are beneficial on the peri-ulcer skin in the presence of wet eczema (Cutting and White, 2002).

Skin assessment

There are a number of factors to which skin may be vulnerable and require protection, namely:

- incontinence (_Figure 5.8_)
- drainage from fistula
- drainage from stoma (_Chapter 7_)
- perspiration (excessive)
- wound exudate
- removal of adhesive products from fragile skin

- sensitivities (allergy or irritant reactions) to products such as skin creams, dressings, adhesives, and incontinence pads (*Figure 5.9*).

Factors that should be considered in relation to skin assessment include:

- skin colour
- texture
- moisture — excess sweating can lead to maceration
- temperature
- sensation.

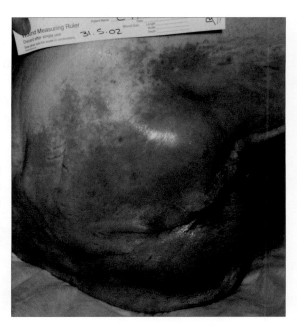

Figure 5.8: The result of incontinence

Neonatal skin requires particular consideration as babies wear nappies (and so have perineal skin exposed to faeces and urine), and may incur wounds such as extravasation injury, intertrigo, abrasions and animal bites (Bale and Jones, 1996), which may lead to maceration.

A scale to measure outcomes of care has been developed using TELER indicators (Treatment Evaluation by Le Roux's method; Le Roux, 1995; Grocott, 1999). This is a unique measuring scale for making and presenting clinical notes on a patient or client to establish the

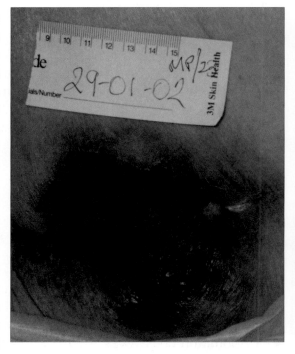

Figure 5.9: A sensitivity to incontinence pads

effectiveness of the treatment or care received. In terms of fluid (exudate) handling of dressings and patient assessment, the WRAP principles (Wound Research for Appropriate Products) are also important to consider (Grocott, 2005).

Wound assessment

Surgical wounds that are created in healthy tissue with limited underlying pathological conditions, and minimal risk of infection, usually heal well and maceration is rarely an issue (White and Cutting, 2003). However, a wound that is healing by secondary intention will produce more exudate, particularly if the wound is heavily colonised with bacteria. The amount of fluid is also influenced by the size and depth of the wound.

Young (1997), and more recently Bentley (2001), have proposed that wound assessment should consider the patient perspective. Russell (2002) proposes a standardised approach to assessment and re-assessment, which includes:

1. The environment.
2. A holistic assessment of the individual.
3. Nutrition.
4. Specific assessment of the wound.
5. Consideration of the skin as a sensory organ.
6. Assessment of the patient's knowledge and understanding of their wound and general condition.

Assessment of exudate will allow a management plan to be instigated.

Peri-wound assessment

The maintenance of good skin condition around fistulae, stomas, and peg sites, requires products that provide skin protection. Assessment approaches and protection of 'at risk' skin have been subject to review (Cameron, 2004; Hampton 2004; Hess 2005) and research (Cameron *et al*, 2005).

Perhaps the best current scheme is that used in Applied Wound Management (Gray *et al*, 2005), where volume and viscosity are presented in a grid, encouraging the practitioner to consider volume as well as viscosity. Traditionally, practitioners have considered exudate in terms of its volume alone; an approach that fails to recognise the potential impact of exudate viscosity which can impact upon the absorptive performance of the dressing. The Wound Exudate Continuum is an assessment tool designed for the assessment of both the viscosity and volume of wounds, and, to rank this combination in terms of clinical significance (Gray *et al*, 2005; White and Gray, 2005).

Maceration in clinical practice

Maceration of the skin and wound bed is caused by prolonged exposure to excess and inappropriately managed exudate. Specific wound types may increase the propensity to macerate because of the pathology or the anatomic location (White and Cutting, 2004); for example:

❖ Leg ulcers

Ulcerated legs have raised intra-capillary pressure resulting from damage to the venous system. This can lead to uncontrolled oedema, which may cause maceration. Exudate management involves a combination of dressings, compression, and limb elevation. The skin directly below the wound is at greatest risk of maceration from leakage. Patients rarely elevate their limbs, especially to the degree recommended.

❖ Pressure ulcers *(Chapter 2)*

Pressure ulcers over the sacrum are particularly at risk of maceration due to urinary incontinence (Collins *et al*, 2002). Skin protection is vital.

❖ Diabetic foot ulcers *(Chapter 3)*

Diabetic foot ulcers may develop into chronic, non-healing wounds. The predominantly neuropathic nature of plantar ulcers, where exudate is in contact with thick callus, makes maceration a real risk.

❖ **Incontinence** (*Chapter 6*)

Faecal or urinary incontinence can cause macera continence assessment should be undertaken to treating where possible. Where treatment is una disposable pads or absorbent disposable pants are

Incontinence can lead to skin breakdown and pressure ulcers. Regular inspection of the skin, the ~~~ or repositioning, transfer techniques and the reduction of shear and friction can, along with a barrier cream (such as Cavilon™ Durable Barrier Cream), assist in protecting the skin.

Secure and effective appliances should be provided for urostomy/ ileostomy. Fistulae should be corrected surgically.

❖ **Burns**

Burns can produce high levels of exudate due to the amount of skin loss (Lamke *et al*, 1997). The barrier is lost and the fluid leaks with the potential colonisation of bacteria to increase vascular permeability.

❖ **Fungating wounds**

Fungating wounds are frequently highly exuding and malodorous. Prevention of maceration is important as it maintains optimal patient comfort and allows maximum choice of dressing (Grocott, 1999; White and Cutting, 2003).

❖ **Stoma sites** (*Chapter 7*)

The peri-stomal area needs careful protection and a good seal with the stoma flange and the skin (White and Cutting, 2003; *Chapter 7*). Effluent from ileostomy sites, in particular, is corrosive to the skin, causing damaging irritant dermatitis reactions (Lyon and Beck, 2001).

❖ **Lymphoedema**

Lymphoedema is due to either increased pressure within the lymphatic an alteration to the lymphatic vascular network. Lymph is high in, which, in combination with fluid, provides a warm, moist environment that can lead to bacterial infections. Skin changes, such as hyperkeratosis, often accompany lymphoedema, and may lead to cracks, fissures or fungal infection.

Professional accountability and legal issues

It is essential for healthcare professionals to recognise the implications of poor exudate management and the subsequent maceration that can develop. There is a need for the practitioner to strive for optimum moisture balance at the wound interface. Consideration should focus on exudate type, volume, patient lifestyle, and location of the wound, as accurate assessment, clear planning and preventative strategies can prevent maceration

Being accountable involves being answerable for decisions that are taken. Accurate and timely record keeping is an integral part of nursing practice (Nursing and Midwifery Council [NMC], 2002). This promotes continuity of care and allows for assessment of the quality of care in partnership with the patient. The patient should be enabled to make an informed choice and, to achieve this, should be supplied with the assessment and the options for treatments, as well as the advantages and disadvantages of treatments.

Post-registration education and practice (PREP) requirements indicate that healthcare professionals should be informed of recent developments within a practice area, so that they can deliver the best possible care for the patient (NMC, 2002).

The prevention of maceration is an essential element of wound care. An educated understanding of the anatomy and physiology of the skin, aetiology of wounds, assessment and knowledge of wound exudate and maceration can improve outcomes for patients. Where maceration does occur, there are evidence-based strategies that can assist in achieving an optimal moist wound environment or providing protection to peri-wound/stoma skin.

Conclusion

It is vital to treat the cause as well as the symptoms in preparing a wound bed to heal. At the same time, it is of extreme importance to understand how the pathology of the wound can effect the surrounding tissues, and how to prevent deterioration of the good skin. This may be achieved with appropriate assessment and careful selection of treatment and dressings.

References

Agren MS (1994) Gelatinase activity during wound healing. *Br J Dermatol* **131**: 634–40

Bale S, Jones V (1996) Caring for children with wounds. *J Wound Care* **5**(4): 177–80

Baatenberg de Jong H, Admiraal H (2004) Comparing cost per use of 3M Cavilon with zinc oxide in incontinent patients. *J Wound Care* **13**(9): 398–400

Bishop SM, Walker M, Rogers AA, Chen WY (2003) Importance of moisture balance at the wound-dressing interface. *J Wound Care* **12**(4): 125–8

Bentley J (2001) Assess, negotiate treat: community prescribing for chronic wounds. *Br J Community Nurs* **6**(6): 302–12

Bowler PG, Duerden BI, Armstrong DG (2001) Wound microbiology and associated approaches to wound management. *Clin Microbiol Rev* **14**(2) 244–69

Bowler PG, Davies BJ (1999) The microbiology of infected and non-infected leg ulcers. *Int J Dermatol* **38**: 573–8

Brew K, Dinakarpandian D, Nagase H (2000) Tissue inhibitors of metalloproteinases: evolution, structure and function. *Biochim et Biophys Acta* **1477**(1–2): 267–83

Cameron J, Powell S (1992) Contact dermatitis: its importance in leg ulcer patients. *Wound Management* **2**(3): 12–13

Cameron J (2004) Exudate and care of the peri-wound skin. *Nurs Standard* **19**(7): 62–6

Cameron J, Hoffman D, Wilson J, Cherry G (2005) Comparison of two peri-wound skin protectants in venous leg ulcers: a randomised controlled trial. *J Wound Care* **14**(5): 233–6

Cameron J, Powell S (1996) Contact kept to a minimum. *Nursing Times Wound Care Supplement* **92**(39): 84–6

Collins F, Hampton S, White RJ (2002) *A–Z Dictionary of Wound Care.* Quay Books division, MA Healthcare Ltd, London

Collier M (2003) The challenge of wound exudate. *Nurs Times* **99**(5): 47–8

Cowley SA, Richardson A, Grocott B et al (2004) WRAP Wound Care Research for Appropriate Products. Position Paper 18. Defining clinical needs for fluid handling devices for chronic wound exudate management. Available online: http://www.66.102.9.104/search?q=cache:PUA_ lSm9vYUJ:www.kcl.ac.uk/wrap/docs/position.pdf+%22wound+maceration %22+prevention&hl=en

Cutting KF (1999) The causes and prevention of maceration of the skin. *J Wound Care* **8**(4): 200–2

Cutting KF (2004) Exudate: composition and functions. In: White R, ed. *Trends in Wound Care, volume III.*Quay Books division, MA Healthcare Ltd, London

Cutting KF, White RJ (2002) Maceration of the skin and wound bed: 1; Its nature and causes. *J Wound Care* **11**(7): 275–8

Cutting KF (2004) Wound exudate. In: White R, ed. *Trends in Wound Care, volume III.*Quay Books division, MA Healthcare Ltd, London

Cutting KF, White RJ (2002) Avoidance and management of peri-wound maceration of the skin. *Prof Nurse* **18**(1): 33–6

Danielsen L (1997) Cadexomer iodine in ulcers colonized by *Pseudomonas aeruginosa. J Wound Care* **6**(4): 169–72

Erikson G, Eklund AE, Kallings LO (1984) The clinical significance of bacterial growth in venous leg ulcers. *Scand J Infect Dis* **16**: 175–80

Goldberg MT *et al* (2000) Oncology-related skin damage. In Bryant R, ed. *Acute and Chronic Wounds.* Mosby, St Louis: 374–7

Gray DG, White RJ, Cooper P (2005) Understanding Applied Wound Management. *Wounds UK* **1**(2): S4–S9

Graham P, Browne L, Capp A *et al* (2004) Randomized, paired comparison of No Sting barrier film versus Sorbolene cream skin care during post-mastectomy irradiation. *Int J Radiat Oncol Biol Phys* **58**(1): 241–6

Grocott P (1999) *The palliative management of fungating malignant wounds.* Wound Care Society Booklet. Wound Care Society, Huntingdon

Grocott P (1998) Exudate management in fungating wounds. *J Wound Care* **7**(9): 445–8

Grocott P (2005) WRAP: defining clinical needs for fluid handling devices. *Wounds UK* **1**(2): 11–19

Hampton S (2004) A guide to managing the surrounding skin of chronic, exuding wounds. *Prof Nurse* **19**(12): 30–2

Hampton S, Collins F (2003) _Tissue Viability a Comprehensive Guide._ Whurr Publications, London

Hansson C, Hoborn J, Moller A, Swanbeck G (1995) The microbial flora in venous leg ulcers without clinical signs of infection. _Acta Dermatol Venereol_ (Stockh) **75**: 24–30

Heggers JP (1998) Defining infection in chronic wounds: methodology. _J Wound Care_ **7**(9): 452–5

Hess CT (2005). The art of skin and wound care documentation. _Adv Skin Wound Care_ **18**(1): 43–53

Hoffman R, Eagle M (1999) The use of proteases as prognostic markers for the healing of venous leg ulcers. _J Wound Care_ **8**(6): 273–6

Lamke L, Nilsson GE, Reithner HL (1997) The evaporative water loss from burns and water permeability of grafts and artificial membranes used in the treatment of burns. _Burns_ **3**: 159–65

Leaper DJ (1994) Prophylactic and therapeutic role of antibiotics in wound care. _Am J Surg_ **167**(1A): 15S–19S; discussion 19S–20S

Le Roux AA (1995) TELER: The concept. _Physiotherapy_ **79**(11): 755–8

Lyon CC, Beck MH (2001) Irritant reactions and allergy. In: Lyon CC, Smith AJ, eds. _Abdominal Stomas and their Skin Disorders._ Martin Dunitz, LondonMulder GD (1994) Quantifying wound fluids for the clinician and researcher. _Ostomy Wound Manag_ **40**(8): 66–9

Neander K D, Hesse F (2003). The protective effects of a new preparation on wound edges. _J Wound Care_ **12**(10): 369–71

Newman D _et al_ (2001) Moisture Control and incontinence management. In: Krasner DL, Rodeheaver GT, Sibbald RG, eds. _Chronic Wound Care: A Clinical Source Book for Healthcare Professionals_, 3rd edn. Wayne PA, Health Management Publications, Inc

Nursing and Midwifery Council (2002) _Nursing and Midwifery Code of Professional Conduct._ NMS, London

Phillips TJ, Al-Amoudi HO, Leverkus M, Park HY (1998) Effect of chronic wound fluid on fibroblasts. _J Wound Care_ **7**(10): 527–32

Rolstad BS, Harris A (1997) Management of deterioration in cutaneous wounds. In: Krasner D, Kane D, eds. _Chronic Wound Care: A Clinical Source Book for Healthcare Professionals_, 2nd edn. Wayne, PA. Health Management Publications, Inc

Russell L (2002) The importance of wound documentation and classification. In: White RJ, ed. _Trends in Wound Care._ Quay Books division, MA Healthcare Ltd, London

Scanlon E, Stubbs N (2004) To use or not to use? The debate on the use of antiseptics in wound care. In: White R, ed. _Trends in Wound Care, volume II._ Quay Books, MA Healthcare Limited, London

Schmidtchen A, Wolff H, Hansson C (2001) Differential proteinase expression by *Pseudomonas aeruginosa* derived from chronic leg ulcers. *Acta Derm Venereol* **81**(6): 406–9

Sibbald G, Cameron J (2001) Dermatological aspects of wound care. In: Krasner DL, Rodeheaver GT, Sibbald RG, eds. *Chronic Wound Care: A Clinical Source Book for Healthcare Professionals*, 3rd edn. Wayne, PA. Health Management Publications, Inc

Thomas S (1997) Assessment and management of wound exudate. *J Wound Care* **6**(7): 327–30

Thompson P (1998) The microbiology of wounds. *J Wound Care* **7**(9): 477–8

Trengove NJ, Stacey MC, McGechie DF, Mata S (1996) Qualitative bacteriology and leg ulcer healing. *J Wound Care* **5**(6) 277–80

Vowden K, Vowden P (2004) The role of exudate in the healing process: understanding exudate management. In: White RJ, ed. *Trends in Wound Care*, volume III. Quay Books division, MA Healthcare Ltd, London

White RJ, Cutting KF (2003). Interventions to avoid maceration of the skin and wound bed. *Br J Nurs* **12**(20): 1186–1203

White RJ, Cooper R, Kingsley A (2001) Wound colonization and infection: the role of topical antimicrobials. *Br J Nurs* **10**(9): 563–78

White RJ, Gray DG (2005) The wound exudate continuum: an aid to wound assessment. *Wounds UK* **1**(2): Suppl S21–S25

Williams C (1998) 3M Cavilon™ No sting Barrier Film in the protection of vulnerable skin. *Br J Nurs* **7**(10): 613–15

Williams C (2001) 3M Cavilon™ Durable Barrier Cream in skin problem management. *Br J Nurs* **10**(7): 469–72

Winter GD (1963) Formation of the scab and the rate of epithelialisation of superficial wounds in the skin of the young domestic pig. *Nature* **193**(4812): 293–4

Wysocki AB, Staiano-Coico L, Grinell F (1993) Wound fluid from chronic leg ulcers contains elevated levels of metalloproteinases MMP-2 and MMP-9. *J Invest Dermatol* **101**: 64–8

Young T (1997) Wound assessment and documentation. *Practice Nurs* **8**(13): 14–9

CHAPTER 6

INCONTINENCE CARE

Sue Bale

Introduction

Urinary incontinence is a common clinical problem affecting many older people. In the USA, it is estimated that between 10%–35% of adults and at least 50% of those cared for in nursing homes (around 1.5 million) are incontinent of urine (Agency for Health Care Policy and Research [AHCPR], 1996). European and UK research supports these USA findings (Durrant and Snape, 2003; Georgiou *et al*, 2001; Hunskaar *et al*, 2004). Bale *et al* (2004) reported the results of a study where 29% of older people cared for in a nursing home were incontinent of urine alone, 65% were doubly incontinent, and 6% were catheterised. Recent audit data shows that at least 50% of nursing home residents in Britain and Northern Ireland suffer from urinary incontinence (Durrant and Snape, 2003); while Georgiou *et al* (2001) report an overall prevalence of 34% in residential homes, 70% in nursing homes, and 71% in long-stay wards. Catheterisation rates were 5% in residential homes, 10% in nursing homes, and 6% in long-stay wards (Georgiou *et al*, 2001). The extent of the problem is thus clearly established.

Chapter 1 describes the structure and functions of the skin, the largest organ in the body, and it is essential that as people get older, clinicians are cognisant of the need to maintain or improve its condition. Healthy, normal skin is the first and best line of defence against the invasion of microorganisms, chemicals, and trauma as the skin is constantly exposed to potential irritants and chemicals, any of which may cause damage (Baranoski and Ayello, 2004). The risk of skin breakdown is also known to increase with age, physical frailty, reduced mobility and incontinence (Springett and White, 2003). Maintenance of the integrity of the skin of the older person is a particular challenge, as people now live for longer, and are continually raising their expectations of health care. In addition,

ped world is experiencing increased numbers of older people
their populations. Davies (1995) reports that despite differing
re systems, country policies for older people are broadly consistent
their targets. The aims of such policies are to maintain older people in
their chosen environment, while promoting autonomy and a meaningful
life (International Association of Gerontology, 1998; DoH, 1998;
Hanford et al, 1999). Nolan (2001) describes global initiatives that aim to
prevent or delay ill health, where nurses are encouraged to be proactive
in improving the health of older people, especially in the community
setting. In the UK, an audit commission review (1999), recommended that
increased attention be paid to the problems of incontinence in patients
cared for in the community. Incontinence has been identified as a factor
that precedes skin damage, and it would seem appropriate that preventing
and managing incontinence should be an important aim of nursing care
(Gray, 2004; Faria et al, 1996; Lyder, 1997; Lyder et al, 1992).

Although a common problem, incontinence carries with it a stigma, as
many with this condition choose not to seek professional help. As a result, it
is both under-diagnosed, under-reported and under-treated (AHCPR, 1996).
A largely hidden problem in the young and independent older persons,
incontinence adversely affects quality of life (Swaffield, 2000). As people
become older, protection of the skin against the effects of incontinence is
of particular importance, and the development of cost-effective, evidenced-
based management strategies should be a priority (Le Lievre, 2001; 2002).

The problem of incontinence

It is expected that adults are in control of bladder and bowel functions,
with incontinence only being tolerated in babies and the very young.
Indeed, much value is often placed on children achieving continence in the
Western world. However, epidemiological research reports that the number
of people experiencing incontinence far exceeds the number that seek
help and advice from healthcare professionals (Swaffield, 1999). Urinary
incontinence is not a disease in its own right, rather symptomatic of a
broad range of underlying conditions. It is most common in older women,
affecting 11.6% of all women included in a postal survey of 22,430 people
(Haggar, 2000). In this survey, stress incontinence and urge incontinence
were significantly increased in parous compared to nulliparous women,
particularly in those who had borne four or more children. Urinary

incontinence in women is commonly caused by constipation and by changes to the vagina and urethra, as a result of decreased levels of oestrogen following the menopause (Swaffield, 2000; Rigby, 2005).

There is some evidence that attitudes towards incontinence are improving. Willis (1996) reports the value of a national awareness campaign by the UK Department of Health and the Continence Foundation in directing people to the appropriate professional services. In addition, the Royal College of Physicians reports that the number of people seeking healthcare advice is increasing (Royal College of Physicians, 1995).

Swaffield (2000) highlights the extent of the problem of incontinence in healthcare institutions and social services facilities. She reports that many surveys have demonstrated high rates of incontinence in these care settings, and argues that this is due to inappropriate assessment and intervention on the part of healthcare professionals. Swaffield also suggests that there is a need not only to identify correctly patients who could be treated, but also to improve public and professional understanding, assessment, treatment and management of incontinence. A recent census of nursing care and care homes highlighted incontinence as extremely prevalent, and caring for incontinence problems accounted for the greatest input in nursing time (Donald *et al*, 2002). Evaluating the impact of a new system for assessing and treating skin for patients with incontinence, Bale *et al* (2004) reported improved patient outcomes on implementation. This focused on the use of a skin care protocol, supported by an educational programme, and used specific skin care products (a skin cleanser, barrier cream and barrier film). Improvements in skin condition with regard to incontinence dermatitis and grade I pressure ulcers were reported, as well as significant savings of staff time and product costs.

Types of incontinence

Urinary incontinence

The most common types of urinary incontinence are stress incontinence, urge incontinence and overflow incontinence:

❖ **Stress incontinence** is the leakage of urine on exertion due to weak urethral spincter and/or pelvic floor muscles (NHS Scotland, 2002).

Failure of the urethral sphincter results from a weakness in the pelvic floor, allowing the urethra to descend and the sphincter to open. This type of incontinence commonly occurs with sudden abdominal pressure on the bladder, usually on coughing, laughing or sneezing.

❖ **Urge incontinence** is the leakage of urine due to uncontrollable bladder spasm (NHS Scotland, 2002). It is caused either by an overactive detrusor function (motor urgency) or by hypersensitivity (sensory urgency). Contraction of the detrusor muscle of the bladder leads to the urge to void — even though only a small amount of urine has collected.

❖ **Overflow incontinence** is caused by urinary retention that arises due to an obstruction (faeces or tumour), an under-active detrusor muscle, or failure of the urethra to open.

Faecal incontinence

Faecal incontinence is far less common than urinary incontinence. Johansen and Lafferty (1996) report faecal incontinence as being especially prevalent in older people and those requiring long-term care. This type of incontinence is typically caused by constipation or faecal impaction, and also by damage to the pelvic floor and anal sphincter.

How incontinence damages skin

The effects of age on the physiology of skin are described earlier (*Chapter 1*). When these are combined with incontinence in the older population, the skin becomes much more vulnerable. Damp skin, caused by exposure to excessive moisture as a result of incontinence, is at risk of loss of barrier function and becomes more vulnerable to shearing forces. In addition, incontinence in old age renders the skin vulnerable to damage, eg. from caustic moisture from urine; stool or frequent washing, all reduce skin tolerance. Skin maceration is a result of prolonged exposure of the skin to excessive moisture from profuse sweating, urinary incontinence, and wound exudate. Cutting and White (2002) describe macerated skin as being a frequent result of urinary incontinence. The literature from 1974 onwards supports a strong relationship between excessive skin moisture and the development of pressure ulcers (White and Cutting, 2004). Older people can experience specific skin pathology with incontinence, namely the adult form of nappy rash is incontinence dermatitis (Le Lievre, 2001).

Incontinence dermatitis

Hampton and Collins (2001) highlight the problem of maceration and associated excoriation as increasing the risk of damage to the skin from friction. As discussed above, patients generally experience urinary incontinence more frequently than faecal incontinence. Fiers (1996) highlights the harmful effects of urinary incontinence on the skin where bacteria and ammonia cause undesirable skin conditions and destructive enzymatic activity is also increased. A combination of urinary and faecal incontinence is most harmful to skin (Leyden *et al*, 1977; Berg, 1986; Kemp, 1994). Urine and faeces together raise the pH of skin and thus increase the activity of harmful proteases and lipases. Andersen *et al* (1994) described this when reporting the results of a study that included healthy human volunteers. They observed that when applied directly onto healthy skin, the digestive enzymes found in faeces caused severe skin irritation. Exposure to excessive moisture increases the permeability of the skin and leads to a reduction of the skin barrier function. Patients in whom the skin barrier function has been disturbed in this way are at risk from developing contact dermatitis, an exogenous eczema, caused by external factors that have either irritated the skin or caused an allergic reaction (Cameron and Powell, 1992). Incontinence dermatitis is an irritant dermatitis, which occurs as a result of high moisture exposure, friction, bacteria and enzymatic activity. Nursing assessment tools and clinical guidelines designed to identify patients at particular risk of skin damage, highlight both urinary and faecal incontinence as contributory factors (AHCPR, 1996).

Why soap and water damage vulnerable skin

When patients experience episodes of incontinence, they are washed to remove the harmful chemicals contained in urine and/or faeces and also to eliminate malodour and promote patient comfort. When patients are incontinent it follows that they are usually washed more frequently. As the skin becomes more alkaline, its permeability to water-soluble irritants increases (Bale *et al*, 2004), thus rendering it more vulnerable to tissue breakdown. If soap and water is used, the pH of skin alters, becoming alkaline instead of acidic, adversely affecting its protective function (Gfatter *et al*, 1997). The pH of normal skin surface is about 5.5, referred to as the 'acid mantle', because at this pH bacterial growth is inhibited as is the action of digestive enzymes (Rippke *et al*, 2002). Kirsner and Froelich (1998) suggest that there is a close relationship between skin surface pH and its bacterial flora of Micrococceae, coagulase negative *Staphylococci, Propionibacterium acnes* and *Propionibacterium granulosum.* Earlier experimental research supports this (Korting *et al*, 1987; Korting and Braun-Falco, 1996). When alkaline soap is used to cleanse the skin, the pH increases so encouraging bacterial growth (Korting and Braun-Falco, 1996; Schmid and Korting, 1995). Surfactants found in soap are irritant, causing alterations in skin barrier properties through swelling and disruption of both its lipid and protein components (Kirsner and Froelich, 1998; Bryant and Rolstad, 2001).

Soap consists of fatty acids or triglycerides and has been used as a cleansing agent for thousands of years. In general use soap is beneficial, Kirsner and Froelich (1998) report the benefits of using soap in health care for infection control, to cleanse skin, and prevent disease. This is not the case for patients who are experiencing incontinence, as soap is alkaline and reduces the thickness of the stratum corneum and emulsifies and removes the protective lipid coating of the skin (Korting and Braun-Falco, 1996). It takes forty-five minutes to restore normal skin pH following washing with soap, and following prolonged exposure, can take nineteen hours. In addition, washing macerated, excoriated skin with soap and water will lead to dryness of the skin by decreasing the natural skin lubricants, so interfering with its water holding capacity (Bryant and Rolstad, 2001).

Why specialised skin care products are better

Specialised skin care products are designed to gently, but effectively, cleanse the skin of adult urine and faeces, while maintaining the acid mantle (AHCPR, 1996). In many Western countries, skin care of patients with incontinence consists of the use of a skin cleanser, followed by skin protection with a barrier preparation (Schuren *et al*, 2005). Jeter and Lutz

(1996) and Whittingham and May (1998) report the benefits of using specialised skin moisturisers when caring for patients with incontinence, as it relieves dryness and protects against excessive moisture and irritants. They report that specialised skin protectants provided better protection against washing than other protectants.

Research has demonstrated the effectiveness of implementing skin care protocols for patients with incontinence. Lewis-Byers *et al* (2002) report the results of a small RCT, where the use of soap and water and a moisturiser was found to be less effective and more time-consuming than using a no-rinse cleanser and a durable barrier cream. Bale *et al* (2004) report similar results, reporting a statistically significant reduction in the incidence of incontinence dermatitis and grade I pressure ulcers in combination with significant savings in staff time and product costs.

The difference between incontinence damage and pressure ulcers

There is increasing recognition that there are many similarities between incontinence damage lesions and superficial pressure ulcers. This can confuse experienced and inexperienced practitioners, as the cause and subsequent treatment of these two skin problems is very different (Defloor *et al*, 2005). It is essential that practitioners are able to assess accurately, so as to treat these skin conditions effectively. Differentiating between these two types of skin damage is more difficult than many practitioners might at first suppose (Defloor *et al*, 2005). By way of providing guidance, these authors offer suggestions for differentiating between incontinence lesions and pressure ulcers (*Table 6.1*).

Defloor *et al* (2005) also provide guidance on identifying patient-related characteristics in order to find out the cause, these include:

- checking the (wound) history in the patient record
- finding out which measures have been taken/what care is provided
- finding out what the skin condition is at different pressure points
- checking whether the movements, transfers and position (changes) of the patient, may have caused the lesion
- finding out whether the patient is incontinent, considering whether the lesion is a moisture lesion or not
- excluding other possible causes.

Table 6.1: Wound-related characteristics (reproduced by kind permission of Defloor and Clark, 2005)

	Pressure ulcer	Moisture lesion	Remarks
Causes	Pressure and/or shear must be present	Moisture must be present (eg. shining, wet skin caused by urinary incontinence or diarrhoea)	If moisture and pressure/shear are simultaneously present, the lesion could be a pressure ulcer as well as a moisture lesion (combined lesion)
Location	A wound not over a bony prominence is unlikely to be a pressure ulcer	A moisture lesion may occur over a bony prominence. However, pressure and shear should be excluded as causes and moisture should be present. A combination of moisture and friction may cause moisture lesions in skin folds. A lesion that is limited to the anal cleft only and has a linear shape, is not a pressure ulcer and is likely to be a moisture lesion. Peri-anal redness/skin irritation is most likely to be a moisture lesion due to faeces.	It is possible to develop a pressure ulcer where soft tissue is compressed (eg. by a nutrition tube, nasal oxygen tube, urinary catheter). Wounds in skin folds of bariatric patients may be caused by a combination of friction, moisture and pressure. Bones may be more prominent where there is significant tissue loss (weight loss)
Shape	If the lesion is limited to one spot, it is likely to be a pressure ulcer. Circular wounds or wounds with a regular shape are most likely pressure ulcers, however, the possibility of friction injury has to be excluded	Diffuse, different, superficial spots are more likely to be moisture lesions. In a kissing ulcer (copy lesion), at least one of the wounds is most likely caused by moisture (urine, faeces, transpiration or wound exudate).	Irregular wound shapes are often present in a combined lesion (pressure ulcer and moisture lesion). Friction on the heels may also cause a circular lesion with full-thickness skin loss. The distinction between a friction lesion and a pressure ulcer should be made based on history and observation
Depth	Partial-thickness skin loss is present when only the top layer of the skin is damaged (grade II). In full-thickness skin loss all skin layers are damaged (grade III or IV). If there is a full-thickness skin loss and the muscular layer is intact, the lesion is a grade III pressure ulcer. If the muscular layer is not intact, the lesion should be diagnosed as a grade IV pressure ulcer	Moisture lesions are superficial (partial-thickness skin loss). In cases where the moisture lesion gets infected, the depth and extent of the lesion can be enlarged/deepened extensively	An abrasion is caused by friction. If friction is exerted on a moisture lesion, this will result in superficial skin loss, in which skin fragments are torn and jagged

Skin assessment and skin care

The ACHPR guidelines for managing patients with urinary incontinence (1996) recommend that: skin is inspected regularly, gently cleansed with a pH-balanced cleansing agent immediately after soiling, absorptive pads and a topical barrier are used to protect the skin from moisture. Recent UK Best Practice Statements (BPS) similarly recognise the need for skin inspection (Nursing and Midwifery Practice Development Unit [NMPDU], 2002); and the need for appropriate skin cleansing (NMPDU, 2005). It is generally considered that assessments should include the following elements:

* Skin condition should be assessed regularly. For the older person with incontinence this may be daily or more frequently. Assessment for tissue damage and the development of a pressure ulcer is needed, as well as assessment for incontinence dermatitis. The EPUAP provides guidance on assessing skin for pressure ulcer development on the web site: www.epuap.org. This contains the PUCLAS Pressure Ulcer Classification training programme designed by Tom Defloor (Defloor and Clark, 2005). It is an interactive programme that has a theoretical page and self-assessment test page, where practitioners can evaluate their knowledge while they study.
* Assess level of continence and treat incontinence appropriately. This may involve adapting patients' physical environment to include providing clothing that can be easily removed, physiotherapy, improving access to toilets, providing walking aides and assistance to access toilets, regular toileting, or provision of commode, and regular cleansing and changing of soiled incontinence aides.
* Skin care: the aim here is to keep the skin clean, dry, and well moisturised to maintain the best barrier possible against skin damage. AHCPR guidelines (1996) and NMPDU (2005) recommend that skin should be cleansed at the time of soiling, as well as at regular intervals. The use of specialised, pH-balanced skin cleansers, the avoidance of damaging soaps, and protecting with skin barriers appropriate to individual patient needs, are all important elements (Baatenburg de Jong and Admiraal, 2004; Schuren et al, 2005). Regimes that include the use of these specialised products have been demonstrated to be effective at improving skin condition for patients with incontinence (Dealey, 1995; Whittingham and May, 1998; Cooper and Gray, 2001; Hampton and Collins 2001; Lewis-Byers et al, 2002; Bale et al, 2004).

...mend:

skin cleanser to effectively remove urine
skin as soon as possible after the soiling has
limit the effects of chemical irritation (AHCPR,
.d skin cleansers have cleansing, emollient,
.deodorant properties that are required to remove
.ne and faeces while maintaining the natural protective
barrı.   .e skin.

❖ Protecting clean skin with a pH-balanced moisturising barrier cream. Dry skin can affect up to 80% of older people; dryness leads to a less pliable stratum corneum that is prone to cracking, flaking and pruritus (Hess, 1997). Specialised barrier creams are designed to protect adult skin from the effects of exudate, urine and faeces, as well as moisturising — so protecting from the effects of skin dryness. Some of these specialised creams are designed to be long-lasting and durable, and applied once a day, provide protection, keeping the skin moisturised.

❖ Extra protection is needed for patients with incontinence dermatitis as the skin is often damaged, oozing, wet and irritated. Film-forming skin protectants incorporate a copolymer that acts as a clear and breathable protective film, which protects against moisture and irritants (Newman *et al*, 1997). Silicone film barriers provide a higher level of protection from the effects of urine and faeces than barrier creams, and their use is recommended to avoid creating or extending skin damage (White and Cutting, 2004). These are applied to the affected area as a clear liquid and allowed to dry, forming a protective film barrier. When patients are incontinent, the area can be cleansed and the film barrier will stay in place, only requiring re-application about every thirty-six hours.

Skin care for patients with both incontinence and wounds

In situations where patients with incontinence also have wounds, excessive exudate can damage the vulnerable peri-wound skin through enzymatic activity and by causing physical damage to the structure of skin. Cutting and White (2002) propose that when patients have existing pressure ulcers, the exudate that drains can cause skin damage by irritating the surrounding skin. In chronic wounds, protease enzymes (present in the exudate), particularly matrix metalloproteases are thought to actively damage healthy skin through their enzymatic action (Chen *et al*, 1992; Trengove *et al*, 1996; Trengove *et al*, 1999; Wysocki *et al*, 1993).

In addition to incontinence, excessive wound exudate can cause physical damage to the structure of the skin. Cutting (1999) describes how the stratum corneum initially absorbs fluid, causing swelling. Further saturation reduces barrier function, leading to skin breakdown. As with urinary incontinence, the peri-wound skin can become macerated due to prolonged contact with the wound exudate.

The patient may complain of burning, stinging and itching of the affected area. Treatment of erythematous maceration may require the application of a topical corticosteroid preparation to reduce the local inflammation prior to the use of a barrier preparation. Creams are easier to apply to wet skin than ointments. A potent, topical steroid should be used for one to two days only and gradually reduced over the next few days. A barrier preparation can then be applied to the peri-wound area as a skin protectant. Various skin barrier preparations are available including ointments, creams (Williams, 2001) and a barrier film that leaves a protective film on the skin surface. The barrier film comes as a spray and also as an impregnated foam on a stick (Williams, 1998). It can be applied to vulnerable skin under adhesive dressings to aid adhesion and prevent trauma on removal.

Conclusion

Incontinence is common and has the potential to damage skin unless precautions are taken. This chapter has outlined its extent and how incontinence damages the skin and affects the quality of peoples' lives. Incontinence remains a taboo subject, where people are reluctant to seek help until their symptoms are extreme (AHCPR, 1996). Research suggests that the embarrassment experienced by patients in discussing their continence needs can be reduced by health professionals being knowledgeable and having information readily available (NHS Scotland, 2002). It is clear that, whenever possible, incontinence should be prevented and treated. However, for many older people who are frail and dependent, incontinence needs to be managed and skin damage prevented by the implementation of skin care regimes that avoid soap and water, using specialised products that protect skin from the harmful effects of urine and faeces.

References

Agency for Health Care Policy and Research (1996) *Urinary Incontinence in Adults: Acute and Chronic Management, Clinical Practice Guideline Number 2* (1996 Update). AHCPR Publication No 96-0682: March 1996

Andersen PH, Bucher, AP, Saeed I, Lee PC, Davis JA, Maibach HI (1994) Faecal enzymes: in vivo human skin irritant. *Contact Derm* **30**: 152–8

Audit Commission (1999) *First Assessment: A Review of District Nursing services in England and Wales.* Audit Commission, London.

Bale S, Tebble N, Jones VJ, Price PE (2004) The benefits of introducing a new skin care protocol in patients cared for in nursing homes. *J Tissue Viability* **14**(2): 44–50

Baranoski S, Ayello EA (2004) Pressure ulcers In: Baranoski S, Ayello EA, eds. *Wound Care Essentials.* Lippincott, Williams and Wilkins, Springhouse, PA

Baatenburg de Jong H, Admiraal H (2004) Comparing cost per use of 3M Cavilon No Sting Barrier Film with zinc oxide oil in incontinent patients. *J Wound Care* **13**(9): 398–400

Berg RW (1986) Aetiology and pathophysiology of diaper dermatitis. *Adv Dermatol* **3**: 75–98

Bishop SM, Walker M, Rogers AA, Chen WYJ (2003) Importance of moisture balance at the wound-dressing interface. *J Wound Care* **12**(4):125–8

Bryant RA, Rolstad BS (2001) Examining threats to skin integrity. *Ostomy Wound Manag* **47**(6): 18–27

Cameron J, Powell S (1992) Contact dermatitis: its importance in leg ulcer patients. *Wound Management* **2**(3): 12–13

Chen WYJ, Rogers AA, Lydon MJ (1992) Characterization of biologic properties of wound fluid collected during early stages of wound healing. *J Invest Dermatol* **99**: 559–64

Cooper P, Gray D. (2001) Comparison of two skin care regimes for incontinence. *Br J Nurs* **10**(6): S6–S20.

Cutting KF (1999) The causes and prevention of maceration of the skin. *J Wound Care* **8**(4): 200–201

Cutting KF, White RJ (2002) Maceration of the skin and wound bed 1: its nature and causes. *J Wound Care* **11**(7): 275–8

Davies B (1995) The reform of community and long-term care of elderly persons: an international perspective. In: Scharf T, Wenger GC, eds. *International Perspectives on Community Care for Older People.* Avebry, Aldershot

Dealey C (1995) Pressure sores and incontinence: a study to evaluate the use of topical agents in skin care. _J Wound Care_ **4**(3): 103–5

Defloor T, Schoonhoven L, Fletcher J, Furtado K, Heyman H, Lubbers M _et al_ (2005) Pressure ulcer classification: differentiation between pressure ulcers and moisture lesions. _EPUAP Review_ **6**(3): 881–5

Defloor T, Clark M (2005) Pressure Ulcer Classification CD. Available online at: http://www.epuap.org (accessed 15 September 2005)

Department of Health (1998) _Modernizing Social Services: Promoting Independence, Improving Protection, Reviewing Standards_. The Stationery Office, London

Donald I, Cope B, Roberts S (2002) Nursing care and care homes — a census view. _J Community Nurs_ **16**(8): 14–15

Durrant J, Snape J (2003) Urinary incontinence in nursing homes for older people. _Age Ageing_ **32**(1): 12–18

Faria DT, Shwayder T, Krull EA (1996). Perineal skin injury: extrinsic environmental factors. _Ostomy Wound Management_ **42**(7): 28–34

Fiers SA (1996) Breaking the cycle: the etiology of incontinence dermatitis and evaluating and using skin care products. _OstomyWound Management_ **42**(3): 33–43

Georgiou A, Potter J, Brocklehurst JC _et al_ (2001) Measuring the quality of urinary continence care in long-term care facilities: an analysis of outcome indicators. _Age Ageing_ **30**(1): 63–6

Gray M (2004) Preventing and managing perineal dermatitis: a shared goal for wound and continence care. _J Wound Ost Cont Nurs_ **31**(1): Suppl: S2–S9

Gfatter R, Hackl P, Braun F (1997) Effects of soap and detergents on skin surface pH, stratum corneum hydration and fat content in animals. _Dermatology_ **195**: 258–62

Haggar V (2000) Strong developments. _Nurs Times_ **91**: 33

Hampton S., Collins F (2001) SuperSkin: the management of skin susceptible to breakdown. _Br J Nurs_ **10**(11): 742–6

Hanford l, Easterbrook L, Stevenson J (1999) _Rehabilitation for Older People: The Emerging Policy Agenda_. King's Fund, London

Hess CT (1997). Fundamental strategies for skin care. _Ostomy Wound Management_ **43**(8): 32–41

Hunskaar S, Lose G, Sykes D, Voss S (2004). The prevalence of urinary incontinence in women in four European countries. _BJU Int_ **93**(3): 324–30

International Association of Gerontology (1998) Adelaide Declaration on Aging. _Aust J Aging_ **17**(1): 3–4

Jeter KF, Lutz JB (1996) Skin care in the frail, elderly, dependent, incontinent patient. _Adv Wound Care_ **9**(1): 29–34

Johanson JF, Lafferty J (1996) Epidemiology of faecal incontinence. The silent afflication. *Am J Gastroenterol* **91**(1): 33–6

Kemp MG (1994) Protecting the skin from moisture and associated irritants. *J Gerontol Nurs* **20**(9): 8–14

Kirsner RS, Froelich CW (1998) Soaps and detergents: understanding their composition and effect. *Ostomy Wound Management* **44**(3A Suppl): 62S–69S

Korting HC, Braun-Falco O (1996) The effect of detergents on skin pH and its consequences. *Clin Derm* **17**: 663–6

Korting HC, Kober M, Mueller M, Braun-Falco O (1987) Influence of repeated washings with soap and synthetic detergents on PM and resident flora on the skin of forehead and forearm. *Acta Derm Venereol* (Stockh) **67**: 41–7

Le Lievre S (2000). Skin care for older people with incontinence. *Elder Care* **11**(10): 36–8

Le Lievre S (2002) An overview of skin care and faecal incontinence. *Nurs Times* **98**(4): 58–9

Lewis-Byers K, Thayer D (2002). An evaluation of two incontinence skin care protocols in a long-term setting. *Ostomy Wound Management* **48**(12): 44–51

Leyden JJ, Katz S, Stewart R, Klingman AM (1977) Urinary ammonia and ammonia producing micro-organisms in infants with and without diaper dermatitis. *Arch Dermatol* **113(12)**: 1678–80

Lyder CH (1997) Perineal dermatitis in the elderly. A critical review of the literature. *J Gerontol Nurs* **23**(12): 5–10

Lyder CH, Clemes-Lowrance C *et al* (1992) Structured skin care regimen to prevent perineal dermatitis in the elderly. *J ET Nurs* **19**(1): 12–16

NHS Scotland (2002) *Continence: Adults with urinary dysfunction best practice statement.* Nursing and Practice Development Unit, Edinburgh

Newman DK, Wallace DW, Wallace J (1997) Moisture control and incontinence management. In: Kranser D, Kane D, eds. *Chronic Wound Care.* 2nd edn. Wayne, PA, Health Management Publications Inc

Nolan J (2001) Improving the health of older people: what do we do? *Br J Nurs* **10**(8): 524–8

Nursing and Midwifery Practice Development Unit (2002) Pressure Ulcer Prevention: Best Practice Statement. NMPDU, Edinburgh. Available online at: http://www.nhshealthquality.org/nhsqis/files/BPSPressureUlcer Prevention.pdf

Nursing and Midwifery Practice Development Unit (2005) The Treatment/ management of Pressure Ulcers: Best Practice Statement. NMPDU, Edinburgh. Available online at: http://nhshealthquality.org/nhsqis/files/BPS %20Management%20Pressure%20Ulcers%20(Mar%202005).pdf

Rigby D (2005) Urinary urge incontinence: causes and management strategies. _Br J Community Nurs_ **10**(4): 174–8

Rippke F, Schreiner V, Schwanitz HJ (2002) The acid milieu of the horny layer: new findings on the physiology and pathophysiology of skin pH. _Am J Clin Dermatol_ **3**(4): 261–72

Royal College of Physicians (1995) _Incontinence: causes, management and provision_. A report from the Royal College of Physicians. RCP, London

Schmid MH, Korting HC (1995) The concept of the acid mantle of the skin: its relevance for the choice of skin cleansers. _Dermatology_ **191**(4): 276–80

Schuren J, Becker A, Sibbald RG (2005) A liquid-forming acrylate for peri-wound protection: a systematic review and meta-analysis (3M™ Cavilon™ No-sting Barrier Film). _Int Wound J_ **2**(3): 230–8

Springett K, White R J (2003). Skin changes in the 'at risk' foot and their treatment. In: White R, ed. _Trends in Wound Care, volume II_. Quay Books, MA Healthcare Limited, London

Swaffield J (2000) Continence. In: Alexander MF, Fawcett JN, Runciman PJ, eds. _Nursing Practice: Hospital and Home, The Adult_. Churchill Livingstone, Edinburgh

Thomas Hess C (1997) Fundamental strategies for skin care. In: Kranser D, Kane D, eds. _Chronic Wound Care_, 2nd edn. Wayne, PA, Health Management Publications Inc

Trengrove N, Langton SR, Stacey MC. (1996) Biochemical analysis of wound fluid from non-healing and healing chronic leg ulcers. _Wound Rep Regen_ **4**: 234–9

Trengove NJ, Stacey MC, MacAuley S (1999) Analysis of the acute and chronic wound environments: the role of proteases and their inhibitors. _Wound Repair Regen_ **7**: 42–52

White RJ, Cutting KF (2004) Maceration of the skin and wound bed by indication. In: White R, ed. _Trends in Wound Care_. Quay Books, MA Healthcare Limited, London

Whittingham K., May S (1998) Cleansing regimes for continence care. _Professional Nurse_ **14**(3): 167–72

Williams C (1998) 3M™ Cavilon™ No Sting Barrier Film in the protection of vulnerable skin. _Br J Nurs_ **7**(10): 44–6

Williams C (2001) 3M™ Cavilon™ Durable Barrier Cream in skin problem management. _Br J Nurs_ **10**(7): 469–72

Willis J (1996) Outreach for prevention. _Nurs Times_ **92**(15): 55–8

Wysocki AB, Staiano-Coico L, Grinnell F (1993) Wound fluid from chronic leg ulcers contains elevated levels of metallproteinases MMP-2 and MMP-9 _J Investigative Dermatol_ **101**: 64–8

CHAPTER 7

STOMA-RELATED SKIN COMPLICATIONS

Angela Vujnovich

Introduction

There are approximately 100,000 people in the United Kingdom living with a stoma (Lee, 2001). Each year in Great Britain, 20,000 new stomas are formed. This figure is made up of 10,000 new colostomies, 8,000 new ileostomies and 2,000 new urostomies (IMS Health Incorporated Group, 2004). Previously, two-thirds of these stomas would have been permanent. As surgery has continued to develop and evolve, it is now estimated that it is an even 50% split between permanent and temporary stomas. Patients may undergo stoma-forming surgery for a variety of reasons. These include:

- cancer of the bowel or bladder
- inflammatory bowel disease
- diverticular disease
- familial adenomatous
- polyposis
- ischaemic bowel
- obstruction
- incontinence
- abdominal trauma
- congenital malformations.

As with any surgery, there is always a risk of complications. With stoma-forming surgery, there is not only an immediate surgical risk such as post-operative bleeding or infection, but also the risk of a stoma-related complication, which can be immediate or delayed. It has been reported that 47% of stoma patients will suffer at least one stoma complication (Lyon and Smith, 2001). Shellito (1998) suggested that the greatest risk of developing a stoma-related complication is usually within the first five years following surgery. Arumugan *et al* (2003) reported that 50% of patients had developed one or more complications within twelve months after stoma-forming surgery.

Stoma-related complications include:

- parastomal hernia
- stoma retraction
- stenosis of the stoma
- prolapse of the stoma
- parastomal granulomas
- mucocutaneous separation.

While these complications are fairly common, by far the most common stoma-related complication is a skin-related one.

A review of the literature will find figures ranging anywhere from 5% (Shellito, 1998) to 42% (Borwell, 1996); with Lyon *et al* (2000) suggesting that 73% of people with a stoma will self-report a skin-related complication.

While a minor skin problem may not at first appear to have any serious consequences, it is important to remember that intact skin is essential for the normal use of a stoma appliance (Smith *et al*, 2002). Any area of skin that has become excoriated, is weeping or bleeding, can cause the stoma appliance to leak. This, in turn, causes the skin to deteriorate further, causing further appliance leaks, hence, the vicious cycle continues. If the patient is experiencing frequent appliance leakage, they will lose confidence in the appliance that they are using which will have a major impact on their activities of daily living and physiological well-being. Patients may report being too scared to leave their house for fear of the appliance leaking.

Skin excoriation can occur at any time and for many reasons (McKenzie and Ingram, 2001). Dermatitis from stoma effluent repeatedly leaking onto the skin is the single most common cause of peristomal skin complications (Lyon and Beck, 2001). Patients who present with a skin complication will usually fall into one of five categories:

- faecal/urine dermatitis
- trauma
- infection
- pre-existing skin conditions
- allergy (Lyon and Smith, 2001).

Within each of these categories there will be different causes. Each will have different signs and symptoms that will affect individual patients in various ways, as well as having different modes of treatment.

Education of the patient with a new stoma in the immediate post-operative phase can minimise the risk of potential skin problems arising (Vujnovich, 2004). A trained stoma care nurse based in the hospital usually undertakes this. However, as most skin complications will develop after the patient has been discharged from hospital, district and practice nurses will encounter people with a stoma in the community.

This chapter will focus on faecal or urinary skin excoriation, as this is the most common cause of stoma-related skin complaints. Trauma and allergy will also be mentioned. Treatment for faecal or urinary skin complaints can be commenced by a healthcare professional in the community with some knowledge of stoma and skin care. In instances where treatment has been commenced with no signs of improvement, the patient should be referred to their stoma care nurse. Skin complaints such as infections and pre-existing skin conditions should be referred to a stoma care nurse or dermatologist, as often the treatment required can impair the adherence of stoma appliances, leading to secondary skin complications.

Faecal or urine dermatitis

Faecal irritant reactions are more common around ileostomies than colostomies, due to the corrosive nature of the effluent. The effluent of ileostomies is strongly alkaline and contains unabsorbed waste products and enzymes that break down protein. Protein is a major constituent of the outermost layers of the skin and protects the skin from harmful substances. The stratum corneum is resistant to quite acidic fluid, but it is more vulnerable to alkaline substances (Stevens and James, 2003). When ileostomy fluid leaks onto the skin, the enzymes break down the protective layers of the skin and cause excoriation.

Urine that is in prolonged contact with the skin will lead to maceration in patients with a urostomy (Collett, 2002). Ideally, urinary pH should be slightly acidic and range between 6–7.5 (Fillingham and Douglas, 1997). An alkaline urinary pH of 7–8 can lead to complications with the peristomal skin and stoma, such as stomal bleeding, ulceration, urinary tract infections, odour and urinary calculi (Fillingham and Douglas, 1997). Eventually, stoma stenosis, pseudoepithelial hyperplasia and hyperkeratosis may occur (Walsh, 1992).

Patient and skin assessment

When first encountering a patient who says that they have excoriated skin, it is important to take a thorough history of the problem. Asking appropriate questions will often give numerous clues as to the cause of their skin complaint (Vujnovich, 2004) (*Table 7.1*).

Table 7.1: History of skin problems	
Questions to ask	Rationale
When did this problem first appear?	Indicates how long the problem has been present
Has the appearance of the excoriation changed?	The excoriation may be improving or worsening, changes may indicate different stages of excoriation
Have you had this problem or any problem with your skin before?	May suggest past history of pre-existing skin problems
What treatment did you try last time or this time?	Previous treatment that may have been effective in the past, may be effective this time
Do you notice leakage at particular times?	Problems may only be reported at particular times (ie. during exercise, at night, when sitting)
What appliance are you using?	Is this appliance appropriate now
Are you using any accessories with your stoma appliance?	Allergies are common to accessories rather then stoma appliances
How many times a day/week do you change your appliance?	May indicate too frequent appliance changes or leaving the appliance in place for too long
How many leaks a week do you experience?	Vicious circle of frequent leaks causing deterioration in skin, causing further leaks
How many times a day do you empty your appliance?	Stoma output may be high, the appliance may get too full before emptying, causing drag on the skin
Has the stoma effluent changed?	Stoma output may have increased, become more loose

All questions should be fully explored to gain a better understanding of the skin complication. Once you have completed taking a history, the next step should be a physical examination of the patient.

Start by looking at the patient's abdomen with the appliance still on. Observe the patient in different positions. Watch how the appliance changes, moves and moulds to the contours of the patient's shape in these different positions. Some appliances may be too rigid for the shape of the patient's abdomen. Skin folds may develop on moving, causing the appliance to lift slightly off the skin, which allows stoma effluent to seep underneath the appliance.

It is then important to watch the patient change their stoma appliance. Pay particular attention to how the patient removes the appliance and how they clean and dry their skin. If the patient is roughly pulling their appliance off, this may cause trauma to the skin; likewise over-vigorous cleaning could destroy the skin.

Once the appliance is off, look carefully at the back of the base plate to assess where any leakage or seepage of effluent has been occurring, subsequently affecting this area of skin. Visible tracks of effluent on the base plate will indicate where stoma effluent has been on the skin.

Now, carefully examine the area surrounding the stoma. The distribution of the excoriation will be determined by the leakage of the stoma effluent on the skin. For the skin to become excoriated it must be in contact with faeces or urine. Pull apart any skin folds to see if the excoriation is present in the folds.

Signs of peristomal skin excoriation:

* Well-defined erythema.
* Oedema may be present.
* Blister formation.
* Areas of denuded skin.
* In severe cases there may be necrosis.
* The patient may describe a burning sensation at the site.
* Itching.

Diagnosing the cause

Your history-taking and physical assessment should have given you clues as to the underlying cause of the skin excoriation. Faecal or urine excoriation will be caused by the following reasons:

- remodelling of stoma
- poorly-sited stoma
- poorly-shaped stoma
- retracted stoma.

Remodelling of stoma

Most newly-formed stomas are oedematous immediately after surgery. Over the first six to eight weeks this oedema will reduce and the stoma will remodel itself. It is important that a new stoma is measured at least weekly in the first two months. This ensures that the appliance aperture is cut to the correct size for the stoma. It is ideal to see 2mm–3mm of skin around the stoma. This provides the skin with maximum protection from the corrosive fluid, but is not too tight for the stoma to be damaged by a tight-fitting appliance. Usually after eight weeks the stoma has stopped remodelling and pre-cut appliances can be ordered.

During your physical examination you may notice an area of excoriated skin directly round the stoma. The area may appear red and angry, areas of skin may be missing and shallow superficial ulcers and dried blood may be present. Patients will complain of pain or a burning sensation at the site. This may be at the circumference of the stoma or to one side. A circumferential ring of excoriated skin would indicate that the patient is cutting the aperture in the appliance too large for the stoma, allowing skin to be exposed to faecal or urinary effluent. If the excoriation is only present in one area around the stoma, usually a crescent shape at the bottom of the stoma, it may be that the patient is not lining up the aperture with the stoma in the middle, but rather slightly off-centre, thereby exposing skin only in one place.

Poorly-sited stoma

All patients having elective surgery that may result in a stoma should be seen pre-operatively by the stoma care nurse for pre-operative education, and to mark the most appropriate site of the stoma. Ideally, the patients belt line should be avoided, the stoma should be located within the abdominal rectus muscle, all creases, skin folds, previous scars should be avoided, and the patient should be able to see the stoma when in various positions such as sitting and standing. However, in emergency situations, pre-operative siting is not always possible and the surgeon is often faced with the dilemma of where to place the stoma. An abdomen may look flat with no skin creases when the patient is on the operating table, but will change dramatically when sitting or standing.

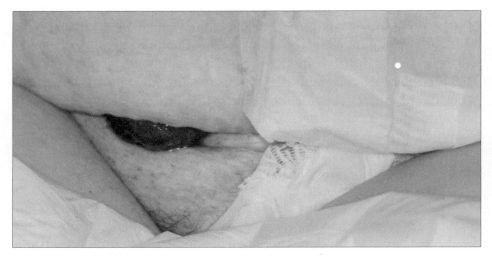

Figure 7.1: Poorly-sited stoma in skin folds

Poorly-shaped stoma

It is ideal for all stomas to have a spout. This is more imperative when dealing with ileostomies and urostomies, rather than colostomies, due to the corrosive nature of the effluent. Spouts encourage the effluent to fall out and into the appliance, rather than trying to track underneath the base plate onto the skin. The optimal shape of an end ileostomy should have a spout long enough to avoid skin excoriation and should point forwards and slightly downwards (Hall *et al*, 1995). In the case of a loop ileostomy, the proximal end where the effluent exits should be everted longer than the distal end (Blackley, 1998). All colostomies should have a spout of a few millimetres (Nicholls, 1996) to avoid excoriation.

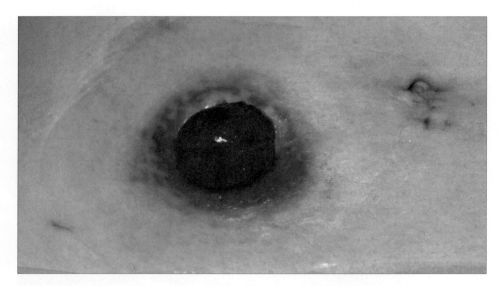

Figure 7.2: Excoriated skin, the circumference of the stoma

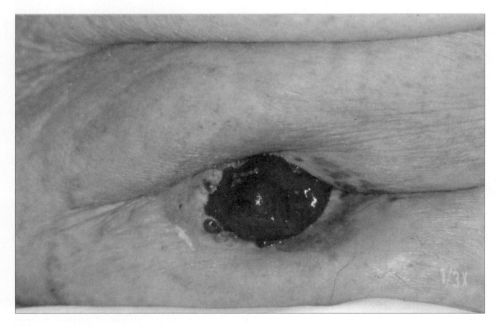

Figure 7.3: Stoma with excoriation tracking along skin crease

Retracted stoma

A retracted stoma is where the stoma has shrunk into a skin fold or dip in the abdomen. Patients with a retracted stoma will usually report frequent leaks, as the output is not flowing into the stoma appliance but leaking underneath the base plate onto their skin. This will cause the skin quickly to become excoriated, leading to further leaks. Retraction can be caused by: technical difficulties at the time of operation in mobilising the bowel to reach the abdominal surface; failure to site the patient pre-operatively so that the surgeon has to guess the most appropriate position of the stoma; or, by weight gain.

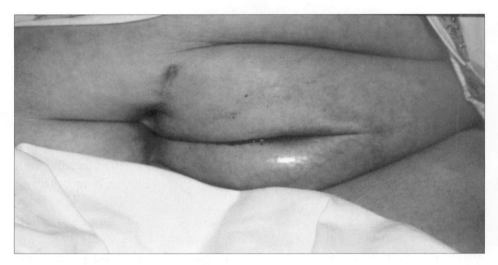

Figure 7.4: Retracted stoma in skin folds

Appliance left on for too long

There may be various reasons why a patient leaves their appliance on for too long. Some patients try to use fewer bags to reduce the need for further prescriptions and charges, while others may think that it only needs to be changed when it begins to leak. Of more concern are the people that find their stoma so abhorrent that they try to ignore it, rather than face changing the appliance. These issues must be explored. Patients that are finding it difficult to come to terms with their stoma will need support and reassurance. Counselling from a trained professional may be required.

High output stoma

The normal output for an ileostomy can range from anywhere between 500mls–1000mls in twenty-four hours. Anything over 1000mls is considered to be a high output. The corrosive nature of ileostomy effluent will damage the skin and erode the stoma appliance quicker. Patients may have to change their appliance more frequently as the appliance will start to erode if left on for long periods.

Treatment of excoriated skin

All excoriated skin should be treated in the same way. Patients should be advised to cleanse the area with warm tap water and dry thoroughly. All stomas should be re-measured using a measuring guide (usually found in the appliance box) to ensure that the aperture of the appliance is cut to the correct size. If the stoma is not round then a template of the stoma shape must be made so that the patient has the correct shape of the stoma to cut the aperture to. It may be beneficial to use a protective barrier such as Cavilon™ No Sting Barrier FIlm (Schuren _et al_, 2005). On application to the skin, Cavilon™ Film forms a waterproof barrier that will act as a protective membrane between the skin and faecal and urinary effluent. The patient should be advised to change the appliance every two days until the excoriation clears up. If the diagnosis is that the patient has been incorrectly measuring the stoma, then this treatment will heal the skin in a matter of days. However, if the stoma is poorly-sited, poorly-shaped or retracted, these measures alone will not stop the excoriation deteriorating or help it to heal. The underlying cause of this excoriation is the fact that the stoma is poorly-sited, poorly-shaped or retracted. The stoma effluent is tracking underneath the appliance causing the leakage, which then excoriates the skin. In these instances, the patient will need assessment from a trained stoma care nurse.

   With modern developments of stoma products, situations like these can be managed conservatively without the need for further surgery to re-site the stoma. Accessories such as paste and seals can be used to build up creases to enable the appliance to stick to a flat surface. Convex appliances raise the profile of the stoma, or the end pointing downwards, by applying a little pressure around the peristomal skin and forcing the stoma out into the appliance. This encourages effluent to fall out into the appliance rather than tracking underneath the appliance onto the skin. A belt can be attached to the appliance to apply further gentle pressure to raise the profile of the stoma and hold the appliance in place. In extreme cases, paste, seals, a convex appliance and a belt may all be needed to manage conservatively the situation and prevent skin excoriation. If it comes to this level of intervention, it may be more appropriate for the stoma to be surgically re-fashioned or re-sited, although this does not guarantee a trouble-free stoma.

If the underlying cause of the excoriation is weight gain on the part of the patient, and their stoma is now retracted, it may be helpful to advise the patient to lose weight. If the stoma has sunk because of the skin folds, it may be necessary to use a convex appliance.

All patients with a high output stoma should be given a barrier protection agent, such as Cavilon™ No Sting Barrier Film, as a prophylactic to avoid skin excoriation, rather than treating it after it has occurred.

Physical irritation

Physical irritation is specifically referring to trauma caused to the skin by factors such as rubbing, pressure, the patient's appliance change technique, or radiotherapy.

Causes of physical irritation include:

- frequent appliance changes
- poor change technique
- treatment of trauma
- radiotherapy and chemotherapy.

Frequent appliance changes

When an appliance is changed too frequently the outer skin cells that provide the skin protection are constantly being stripped off. The skin will have a similar appearance to excoriation caused by effluent leaking onto the skin. It will appear excoriated which may be weeping or bleeding. Areas of skin may be denuded or ulcerated.

Poor change technique

Patients should always be observed changing their appliance to assess their technique (Myers, 1996). Patients may strip their appliance off their abdomen as quickly as possible without supporting the skin. Vigorous rubbing of the skin when cleaning to ensure that all traces of effluent are removed, can also lead to damage. Some patients may have difficulty in lining up the aperture with the stoma, and may be placing it off-centre, exposing the skin to effluent on one side.

Treatment of trauma

There are many different recommendations as to the frequency of appliance changes. Drainable, one-piece appliances or the base plates of two-piece appliances can be changed anywhere from every day to every four days. The average wear time is two to four days (Allen, 1998). If the peristomal skin is in excellent condition, the patient can decide what is the best routine for them. As long as their skin stays in perfect condition, then this is acceptable. However, if they leave their appliance on for several days and their skin begins to deteriorate, they must change their appliance more frequently. For colostomists, it is suggested that they should change their one-piece closed appliance as necessary (Black, 2000), which may be once or twice, daily depending on their output.

A careful assessment must be taken to understand why the appliance is frequently being changed. It may be as simple as the appliance being inappropriate for the stoma effluent, and changing to a more appropriate one would solve this problem. On questioning, some patients will report feeling dirty with faeces sitting in the appliance on their abdomen and they only feel clean when they change the appliance. In these cases, patients require support and advice. Explain to the patient the damage that frequent appliance changes or over-vigorous removal or cleaning and drying does to their skin, by repeatedly removing its protective layers. Patients should be encouraged to gently remove their appliance using one hand to pull the appliance, while the other supports the skin. The patient should demonstrate placing the new appliance in place. Two-piece appliances, where the base plate can be left in place for several days, and the patient can change the bag as needed, will allow the skin to repair itself in-between base plate changes. Patients who experience difficulty lining the aperture with the stoma may find a mirror useful, or a two-piece appliance where they can line the aperture and the stoma up and then clip the bag in place.

Radiotherapy and chemotherapy

Skin problems related to radiotherapy and chemotherapy are relatively uncommon. Often the most common side-effect after chemotherapy and radiotherapy is diarrhoea, which can lead to appliance leakage problems and excoriated skin. When patients are experiencing diarrhoea during the course of their treatment, drainable appliances or a two-piece system (where the base plate can be left in place for several days but the bag changed as needed) should be used while the diarrhoea persists.

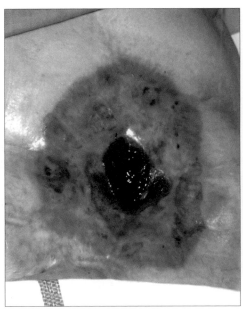

Figure 7.5: Excoriation around the stoma. Note the ulcers directly under the stoma, and to the left and right, caused by over-frequent appliance removal and over-vigorous cleaning to the area. The stoma is also flush with the skin — potentially causing effluent leakage onto the skin

The severity of skin reactions after radiotherapy will depend on the total dose of radiation, the size of the area being treated, and the condition of the skin before commencing radiotherapy. Skin breakdown is most likely to occur in moist areas, skin folds, such as the groin, or in areas of recent surgery, such as the perineal region after an abdominal resection (McGrath and Fulham, 2004)

Skin damage following radiotherapy can be classified as:

* **Erythema** — skin becomes pink, dry and itchy, may have a rash-like appearance or spots, and feel hot, and appears similar to sunburn. Occurs two to three weeks after commencing radiotherapy and resolves two to three weeks after stopping therapy.
* **Dry desquamation** — characterised by dry, flaky, superficial skin loss which is often itchy It is often the precursor of moist desquamation, especially if onset is early in treatment. Occurs two to three weeks after commencing therapy.

* ❖ **Moist desquamation** — skin blisters and sloughs off exposing the dermis. Raw skin may be apparent and bleeding may occur. Exudate may be serous, white, yellow or green.
* ❖ **Necrosis** — this rarely occurs (Faithful, 2001).

In some cases, patients can develop stomatitis when receiving some chemotherapy agents. These include 5-flurouracil, methotrexate, doxorubicin, bleomycin and mitomycin C. The stoma can become oedematous and inflamed. This will not cause the patient any pain, as the stoma has no nerves. Patients should be advised that they might need to adjust the aperture of their appliance to fit the oedematous stoma correctly (Porrett and McGrath, 2005).

Prevention and treatment

Any patients undergoing radiotherapy should seek advice about skin care from the centre providing their treatment. Different centres will have varying recommendations for prevention of damage. Patients should be advised to wash the skin within the treatment area with a mild soap. Moisturising creams should be applied, although alcohol, petroleum, lanolin (Korinko and Yurick, 1997), and metallic-based creams, such as zinc (Lyon and Smith, 2001), should be avoided. Moisturising cream will hydrate the skin. To help soothe the erythema the moisturiser may be placed in the fridge before use. Creams should not be applied within two hours prior to treatment. If patients need to shave their abdomen so the stoma appliance adheres to the skin, they should be advised to use an electric razor rather than a wet razor while receiving radiotherapy. Perfumed products should not be used in the treatment area. Loose clothing, preferably made from natural fibres, should be worn to prevent friction over the area. Any exudate should be blotted dry with sterile gauze. Moist desquamation should not be routinely cleaned unless there is evidence of infection. Trauma of repeated cleaning will increase desquamation and damage granulating tissue.

Allergy

It is important to mention allergy, as most patients will report that their excoriated skin is due to an allergy to their appliance. A true allergy to a stoma appliance is rare and only accounts for 0.6% of stoma-related skin problems (Lyon and Beck, 2001). Suspected skin allergy from stoma products can be broken down into two categories; namely, an allergy to:

- the appliance
- accessory products.

Assessment

Signs and symptoms of skin allergy include:

- erythema
- margins are indistinct and blurred and may spread beyond the area of the appliance
- blister formation
- papules and vesicles often seen
- lesions may become painfully eroded and crusted
- itching.

When examining the skin it is important to look at the distribution of the excoriation on the skin surrounding the stoma. This will often give the best clue as to the cause of the dermatitis. The skin must be in contact with the appliance to develop an allergic reaction to a stoma appliance. If the patient has skin creases, it is important to pull them apart to look for excoriation. If there is excoriation in the creases, it is likely that faeces or urine are tracking along these creases causing the excoriation. If the skin crease shows no signs of excoriation, an allergy may be the cause of the excoriation. While patients can develop an allergy to stoma appliances, it is more common to develop an allergy to a stoma accessory, such as a fragranced stoma bag deodoriser. In several European studies, fragrances have been demonstrated to be second only to nickel as a cause of allergic contact dermatitis (Lyon and Beck, 2001). It is essential to watch the patient do a complete appliance change. The patient may be using potentially irritant substances, such as a deodoriser, perfumed cleansers, or medicated wipes.

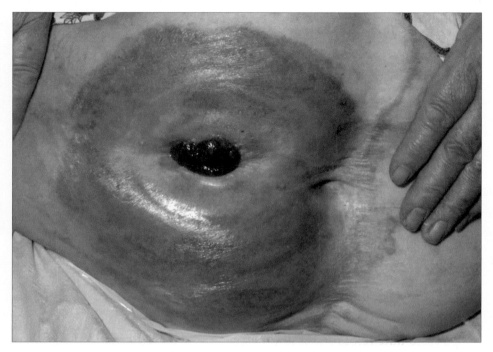

Figure 7.6: Allergy to a stoma appliance

Treatment

Patients should be advised to wash their skin with lukewarm tap water. Perfumed products should be avoided and the use of barrier preparations should only be used if advised by a clinician who has experience in the field of stoma and skin care. Any accessories the patient is using should be stopped immediately.

If an allergy to an appliance is diagnosed, the patient should change the type of appliance to one with a different adhesive, flange or wafer. True allergic dermatitis will resolve when the patient is no longer exposed to the allergen (Lyon and Beck, 2001). The application of a topical steroid to the allergy may hasten its resolution.

Testing for allergy

If an allergy is suspected, a usage test can be tried. Usage testing involves the patient placing the same appliance and any accessories they may be using on the opposite side of their abdomen to their stoma. These will be left on for several days to see if any rash develops. This test will only demonstrate that the patient is sensitive to some component of their stoma products. Further investigations may be required.

Patients requiring patch or prick testing should be referred to a specialist dermatology department with experience in performing this test (Lyon and Beck, 2001). An allergy to a stoma appliance or accessory can be confirmed with a positive patch test. Appliance manufacturers are often willing to give information about compounds used in their products so that the source of the allergy can be identified and avoided in future product usage (Lawson, 2003).

Conclusions

Skin problems are common among patients with a stoma. Patients may develop a skin problem for a variety of reasons, many of which are beyond their control. Careful and thorough history-taking will often give clues as to the cause of the problem. Combine this with a careful, physical examination and a correct diagnosis can usually be swiftly made. Simple measures to treat skin excoriation can be commenced by healthcare professionals with a basic knowledge of stoma and skin care. In some cases, patients may need to be referred to a trained stoma care nurse for specialist advice and treatment regarding stoma appliances.

References

Allen S (1998) Ileostomy. *Prof Nurse* **14**(2): 107–12
Arumugan PJ, Bevan L, MacDonald L, Watkins AJ, Morgan AR, Beynon J, Carr ND (2003) A prospective audit of stomas, analysis of risk factors and complications and their management. *Colorectal Dis* **5**(1): 49–52

Black P (2000) *Holistic Stoma Care*. Baillière Tindall, China

Blackley P (1998) *Practical Stoma Wound and Continence Management*. Research Publications Pty Ltd, Australia

Borwell B (1996) *Managing stoma problems*. Professional Nurse Wallchart. MacMillan Magazines

Collett K (2002) Practical aspects of stoma management. *Nurs Standard* **17**(8): 45–52

Faithful S (2001) Radiotherapy. In: J Corner, C Bailey, eds. *Cancer Nursing: Care in context*. Blackwell Science, Oxford: 222–61

Fillingham S, Douglas J (1997) Urological Nursing. 2nd edn. Baillière Tindall, London

Hall C, Myers C, Phillips RKS (1995) The 554 ileostomy. *Br J Surg* **82**: 1385

IMS Health Incorporated Group (2004) *New Patient Audit*. IMS Hospital Group, London

Korinko A, Yurick A (1997) Maintaining skin integrity during radiotherapy. *Am J Nurs* **97**: 40–4

Lawson A (2003) Complications of Stomas. In: Elcoat C, ed. *Stoma Care Nursing*. Hollister, London

Lee J (2001) Common stoma problems: a brief guide for community nurses. *Br J Community Nurs* **6**(8): 407–13

Lyon CC, Smith AJ, Griffiths CEM, Beck MH (2000) The spectrum of skin disorders in abdominal stoma patients. *Br J Dermatol* **143**(6): 1248–60

Lyon CC, Beck MH (2001) Irritant reactions and allergy. In: Lyon CC, Smith AJ, ed. *Abdominal Stomas and their Skin Disorders: An atlas of diagnosis and management*. Martin Dunitz Ltd, London

Lyon CC, Smith A (2001) *Abdominal Stomas and their Skin Disorders: An atlas of diagnosis and management*. Martin Dunitz Ltd, London

McGrath A, Fulham J (2005) Understanding chemotherapy and radiotherapy for the individual with a stoma. In: Porrett T, McGarth A, eds. *Stoma Care*. Blackwell Publishing, Oxford

McKenzie FD, Ingram VA (2001) Dansac invent convexity in the management of flush ileostomy. *Br J Nurs* **10**(15): 1005–9

Myers C (1996) *Stoma Care Nursing: A patient-centred approach*. Arnold, London

Nicholls RJ (1996) Surgical Procedures. In: Myers C, ed. *Stoma Care Nursing: A patient-centred approach*. Arnold, London

Schuren J, Becker A, Sibbald RG (2005) A liquid film-forming acrylate for peri-wound protection: a systematic review and meta-analysis (3M™ Cavilon™ No Sting Barrier Film). *Int Wound J* **2**(3): 230–8

Shellito P (1998) Complications of abdominal stoma surgery. *Dis Colon Rectum* **41**(12): 1562–72

Smith AJ, Lyon CC, Hart CA (2002) Multidisciplinary care of skin problems in stoma patients. *Br J Nurs* **11**(5): 324–30

Stevens P, James P (2003) Anatomy and physiology associated with stoma care. In: Elcoat C, ed. *Stoma Care Nursing.* Hollister, London

Walsh BA (1992) Urostomy and urinary pH. In: Fillingham S, Douglas J, eds. *Urological Nursing.* 2nd edn. Baillière Tindall, London

Porrett T, McGrath A (2005) *Stoma Care.* Blackwell Publishing, Oxford

Vujnovich A (2004) Peristomal faecal/urine dermatitis and allergy. *Gastrointestinal Nurs* **2**(5): 25–31

CHAPTER 8

NEONATAL SKIN CARE

Valerie Irving

The skin of a newborn infant will differ in structure and appearance, depending on the gestation at birth.

At term (thirty-seven-plus weeks' gestation), the epidermal layers are similar to, but only half as thick as, that found in an adult. The stratum corneum, which gives the skin its barrier function (*Chapter 1*), rapidly matures in the last few weeks before birth. The dermis is 2mm–4mm thick, only half that of adult skin. Following a period of development at birth, the dermis remains constant for the first year of life.

The subcutaneous fat layer is usually well-developed in the term infant, and it is this layer which gives the skin its pink appearance.

At thirty-three weeks' gestation, the layers of the epidermis are fully formed and the skin is considered to be functionally mature. The junction between the epidermis and the dermis is still fragile, and this increases the risk of damage from friction or shearing forces. The subcutaneous layer is well-established and beginning to thicken at this stage of development.

At thirty weeks' gestation, the stratum corneum is only two to three cell layers thick, providing very limited barrier function: an important factor to consider when planning care. However, the surface of the skin is covered with vernix caseosa, composed of sebum from the sebaceous glands. This is thought to help maximise barrier function, as well as protecting the skin from maceration from the amniotic fluid. At this stage of development, the dermis is very oedematous and this may put pressure on the immature capillaries which supply the epidermis, reducing effective oxygenation and making it more susceptible to pressure injuries. The contours of the epidermal/dermal junction (rete pegs) are beginning to become more evident with rete ridges increasing in size (Rudy, 1991).

The skin of infants born at the edge of viability (twenty-four weeks' gestation) has a reddish appearance due to the lack of subcutaneous fat, therefore, the dermis lies directly on top of the muscle tissue. The veins can be easily seen and the surface of the skin has a glistening appearance which is due to the high transepidermal water loss (Rutter, 1996). The stratum corneum is hardly evident and so there is no barrier function to the skin at this stage of development.

Transepidermal water loss

If the barrier function of the skin is compromised, there are severe consequences for the immature infant. Below thirty weeks' gestation, skin water loss could be as high as $65g/m^2/hr$, or, between 85–110mls/kg/day (Harpin and Rutter, 1983).

Nursing the infant under a radiant heater increases the potential for dehydration and fluid imbalance to occur. However, Harpin and Rutter (1985) found that by introducing humidity into the incubators, there was decreased water loss from the skin through evaporation. Modern incubators are double-walled and are able to provide humidity under sterile conditions which reduces the risk of *Pseudomonas aeruginosa* bacterial contamination which was a serious problem at the time of their study (Kuller, 1995).

As the skin responds to the change of environment from the fluid-filled uterus to the atmospheric (gaseous) ex-uterine one, there is a rapid maturation of the barrier function. Harpin and Rutter (1985) found that after two weeks of life, skin water loss had reduced to that of adult levels.

The infant born before the skin is functionally mature (thirty-three weeks' gestation) should be nursed in an humidified environment as temperature control is also improved (as heat loss through convection is reduced), and this has an ongoing positive affect on the general condition (Rutter and Hull, 1979). The maximum humidity constantly achievable is about 90%, and, at this level, water loss through the skin is virtually nil. It is important to ensure that condensation is not allowed to build up on the inside of the incubator canopy, as this has a cooling effect on the infant.

There has been much debate concerning the use of emollients applied to the skin to reduce transepidermal water loss. Early studies looked at the use of a paraffin mixture and, although it did reduce the levels by 40%–60%, it did not help maintain the body temperature (Rutter and Hull, 1981). The effects of a preservative free topical ointment (Aquaphor®, Biersdorf), applied twice daily to pre-term infants nursed under infra-red heaters, have been investigated (Nopper *et al*, 1996). They showed that the trans-epidermal water loss was reduced by 67% within thirty minutes of the application, and was still 34% less than the pre-application loss six hours later. There was no evidence of any toxic reactions to the product when used in this population group which, due to their immaturity, have increased potential for percutaneous absorption of any product applied to the skin.

This product is not available in the UK and the use of a controlled humidified environment is the preferred method, as the use of paraffin-based products leaves the skin unsuitable for some monitoring devices.

Absorption of chemicals

If the barrier function is reduced there is also the potential for any chemicals applied to the skin to be absorbed. In the late 1970s, studies showed that standard 3% hexachlorophene liquid soap used for washing newborn infants for only three to five days resulted in significant blood levels of the compound (West *et al*, 1981). Hexachlorophene was known to be neuro-toxic to animals, but this fact was not widely disseminated and so its potential to cause similar brain damage in infants was not appreciated. Subsequently, many infants died following the use of baby powder contaminated with hexachlorophene, with the most premature infants showing the greatest central nervous system damage.

Topical iodine-based products used for skin cleansing have caused transient hypothyroidism in pre-term infants (Linder *et al*, 1997) and, although the blood levels return to normal, the use of this solution as a routine preparation should be avoided.

Alcohol-based products have been reported to cause haemorrhagic skin necrosis in pre-term infants when there has been prolonged contact, with a subsequent increase in the blood ethanol levels (Harpin and Rutter, 1992; Watkins and Keogh, 1992). If it is felt to be absolutely necessary to use alcohol as a dilutent, contact with the skin should be for the minimum recommended period and the solutions washed off using sterile water. Any spillage onto sheeting should be removed immediately and replaced with dry contact material.

Chlorhexidine in the aqueous form has been used for many years and, although it has the potential to be absorbed when used on the pre-term infant, it does not appear to cause any adverse effects.

Bathing

At birth, the skin surface of a term infant has a pH of 6.34 and, over the next three to four days, this falls to an average of 4.95 reflecting the development of the 'acid mantle' that protects the skin against microbes (Lund, 1999). For the pre-term infant, this process may take up to three weeks and any procedure which interrupts the reducing pH leaves the skin susceptible to excessive bacterial colonisation. Bathing the infant using even the mildest soap can have a drying effect on the skin, and the added dyes and perfumes can cause irritation. The acid mantle can take up to one hour to be restored following use of an alkaline soap, so plain water is sufficient to wash the infant for the first two to three weeks of life until the skin matures. After that, bathing using soap products more than two to three times per week is unnecessary. The use of antimicrobial products for bathing does not give any long-term protection and is not beneficial due to the increased potential for percutaneous absorption.

Nappy rash

The pH of the skin which has been in contact with urine alters from acid to alkaline (ie. from pH 5.0. to over 7.0), this activates the enzymes, protease and lipase, and this can start breaking down the stratum corneum — leading to nappy rash. Prevention is achieved by the use of highly absorbent gel-cored nappies, which draw the urine away from the skin surface. Thick application of any barrier product can result in the urine being left in contact with the skin beneath it, preventing the nappy from being fully effective.

Infants who are recovering from neonatal abstinence syndrome, or those with malabsorption conditions, are at greater risk from nappy rash as the rapid movement of the stools through the small bowel results in a higher pH than normal. Preventative action should be taken in this group of infants by applying a barrier product, such as Cavilon™ (3M) (Schuren *et al*, 2005), to the intact skin on the buttocks, and increasing the frequency of nappy changing. Should the skin in the nappy area break down, consider alternative barrier treatment. Application of a pectin-based product, Orabase® (ConvaTec), or a hydrocolloid-based product, Granuflex Paste® (ConvaTec) is effective at protecting the area from further injury while allowing the damaged area to heal. The stools can be wiped away from the paste, which does not need to be removed, thus reducing the risk of causing further trauma to the area. Leaving the buttocks exposed is not an effective option and only causes more interventions due to the frequency of loose stools; and the infant is less likely to settle due to the lack of comforting boundaries.

Pre-term infants are susceptible to fungal infections due to _Candida albicans_ as a result of opportunist infection following antibiotic therapy, and the warm moist environment in which they are nursed. The skin, where infection is suspected, should be sent for culture and sensitivity to confirm diagnosis. While awaiting results, a suitable anti-fungal regime, such as nystatin, should commence, with both oral medication and topical ointment being prescribed.

With the pre-term infant, there is no advantage in impregnated wipes over the use of plain water for nappy care, as this practice exposes the skin to unnecessary chemicals. In the first month of life, the average neonate is exposed to up to sixty-six different chemicals from skin care products alone (Malloy-McDonald, 1995); all of which have the potential to be absorbed and cause toxicity.

Use of emollients

The use of emollients such as Aquaphor® or petroleum jelly to reduce transepidermal water loss has been well-documented (Pabst _et al_, 1999; Horii and Lane, 2001). These products can be used at a later date to prevent or reduce excessive dryness of the skin, and to prevent the formation of cracks or fissures. Emollients should not be used routinely as they can alter the pH of the skin and have the potential to be absorbed. However, the incidence of nosocomial infections in emollient-treated groups has been found to be less than in the non-treated groups (Nopper _et al_, 1996). A Cochrane Review (Connor _et al_, 2004) of the use of emollient ointment for preventing infection in pre-term infants concluded that they should not be routinely used due to the increased risk of coagulase negative Staphylococcal infection.

Any cream or emollient which is essential must be non-perfumed, without dyes, and preferably without preservatives; as all are known to cause drying and skin irritation in this patient group and must be supplied in single patient containers to prevent cross-infection. In practice, E45 (Crookes) cream is an effective product and parents can be encouraged to apply this as part of their involvement in care provision.

Epidermal stripping

Epidermal stripping is caused by the inappropriate use of tape or adhesive products, when the bond between the product and the epidermis is stronger than the bond between the epidermis and the dermis. The connecting fibrils are fewer in number, and more widely spaced in the pre-term infant (*Chapter 1*). It also occurs when there is undue friction between the infant's skin surfaces, and if there has been inappropriate handling.

The Molloy Protocol was one of the first published sets of guidelines to support nursing care for infants under 1kg. A national survey showed that compromised skin integrity was <90% (Perrez-Woods and Malloy, 1992).

This protocol forms the basis of skin care practices today, and recommends that all tapes need to be evaluated before use to establish an actual need for the product as well as the type and amount required. Tape can be backed with cotton wool to reduce the adhesive properties, or placed back to back to completely prevent any contact with it. A protective, thin hydrocolloid dressing (Duoderm®, ConvaTec) can be used between the skin and the adhesive product; this would remain *in situ* should the product need replacing or re-siting, thus preserving the skin beneath. Monitoring probes could be placed in a 'keyhole' cut into a circular patch of the thin hydrocolloid, and tape applied over the top to secure them. Pieces can be cut into 'Cs' and used around the umbilical stump to attach any tape used as 'bridges' to help secure umbilical arterial or venous catheters in place. Pieces can be applied to the cheeks to attach naso-gastric feeding tubes or oxygen cannulae both to prevent tape damage and reduce pressure. It is important that the thin hydrocolloid is removed using the horizontal stretch method to prevent it causing damage to the delicate skin.

Bonding agents should not be used, as these will increase the risk of epidermal stripping. Also, solvents, because of their potential for further skin damage and the risk of toxicity, should not be used to remove any adhesive products.

If unsettled or agitated, infants can damage their skin from friction against sheeting or other skin surfaces. Care must be taken to nurse on soft sheeting which has been washed with non-biological, non-perfumed products. The use of suitably sized 'nests' and well-positioned bumpers to create boundaries will give a sense of security and may help to reduce the potential for damage, although considered to be more commonly used as developmental care aids.

Skin damage can also be caused by inconsiderate handling or by poorly positioning of monitoring or diagnostic equipment. All staff who are involved in the care of these infants should have a comprehensive education package to increase their awareness, and parents/family members should have a similar package, appropriate to their level of understanding.

The use of sterile clear film dressings for securing IV cannulae in place was recommended over twenty years ago (Smith, 1985), as these give an unrestricted view of the insertion site and surrounding area for early detection of displacement, detachment, phlebitis, infiltration or extravasation. More recently, this has been supported by Bravery (1999) and the Infection Control Nurses Association (ICNA, 2001) and has been adopted as 'Best Practice' by the North West Neonatal Clinical Practice Benchmarking Group. Current products suitable for neonatal use are Tegaderm™ (3M) or Opsite IV® 3000 (Smith and Nephew); however, these products have the potential themselves to cause epidermal stripping if not removed carefully using the horizontal stretch method.

The use of a non-alcohol based skin protective barrier (Cavilon™, 3M) has been evaluated when used underneath these products; there was no visible skin damage when these were removed even on the most premature infant (Irving, 2001). Further studies are needed to establish the percutaneous absorption and potential toxicity of this product, as the manufacturer does not currently recommend its use in infants <30 days.

Hydrogel-based electro-cardiograph electrodes should be used for monitoring purposes as these will not cause skin damage on removal, even on the skin of the most vulnerable infant.

Pressure damage

The typical areas for damage due to pressure are rarely involved in the pre-term infant due to the large surface area to weight ratio and the relative ease of ensuring position changes. However, extremely ill, unstable infants who are hypotensive, hypovolaemic, or requiring inotropes, are potentially at greater risk. The most common areas for pressure damage are the tops and lobes of the ear and the occiput. Prevention by frequent repositioning (three- to four-hourly) must be counterbalanced against any deterioration in condition due to this handling. The use of peanut-shaped pillows, overlays, ie. Spenco incubator pads and gel-filled mattresses can help reduce the risk, but cannot replace good nursing care and careful vigilance.

As described above, pressure caused by catheters or drains can be reduced by the use of a thin hydrocolloid.

Monitoring devices, such as saturation probes, can also cause pressure damage and require careful positioning with non-constrictive velcro wraps, and frequent repositioning, dependent on the individual infant's condition.

Extravasation injuries

Extravasation is the non-intentional leaking of a vesicant solution into the surrounding tissue which results in cell death and tissue necrosis (Gault, 1993). This may be due to the toxic effect of the fluid itself, the irritant nature of low or high pH of the fluid, the increased pressure of the infused fluid on the blood vessels (reducing the circulation to the area), or the change in the osmotic equilibrium between the extra- and the inter-cellular fluids (Gault, 1993).

These are, without doubt, the most serious of all the iatrogenic injuries sustained as the resultant scarring will be a lifelong reminder of the incident. Pre-term infants are more susceptible to such injuries as they require a prolonged period of administration of parenteral nutrition, which is very irritant to veins until enteral feeds are established. If born before thirty weeks' gestation, there is little or no subcutaneous fat layer, and any tissue damage will involve the muscle layer. The median lifespan of a neonatal cannula is only thirty-one hours (Hecker, 1993), and any damage may become obvious immediately the solution is administered, ie. as a bolus or some time after the cannula has been removed.

Ideally, all such injuries could be prevented if peripherally-inserted central catheters were always used to administer these highly irritant solutions. However, due to the physical size of the infant, their unstable condition, or systemic sepsis, it is not possible in every case. In these circumstances, and when administering bolus antibiotics or other medication, peripheral intravenous cannulae are used and require careful monitoring of the site and surrounding area. There is no specific neonatal tool for assessing IV site patency, with units basing their observations on modified adult tools (Jackson, 1998; Intravenous Nurses Society [INS], 2000), with hourly observations recorded and acted upon if signs of blanching or discolouration are found. At the earliest sign of infiltration or extravasation, the cannula must be removed and re-sited.

At present, there is no universal, national or regional agreement on the best practice for managing extravasation injuries, but the use of hydrocolloids and hydrogels has been shown to be effective, following the principles of moist wound healing (Winter, 1962).

Management of wounds

The ideal dressing for neonatal wounds is one which can be cut to size and is effective while in a humidified environment.

The use of a hydrocolloid wound contact material has been shown to be beneficial in the pre-term infant (Young *et al*, 1996). The relatively small sizes required means that the dressing can be overwhelmed by the level of the exudate and may require daily changes which is not ideal. When this phase is passed, the hydrocolloid has a wear time of seven days making it both cost-effective and an efficient wound contact material.

The use of a hydrogel has been reported for the treatment of infant skin injuries (Thomas, 1987). Its use is limited to dorsal limb injuries as, due to the high ambient temperature of the incubators and the clinical environment, the gel had to be placed in a plastic bag to prevent it drying out in a matter of hours. This means that the entire limb has also to be treated, potentially leading to maceration of the surrounding area. Although the digits can move freely in the gel, the overall weight required means that a small infant cannot move the limb itself, and the bagged gel may have to be supported with a splint.

With the ongoing development of wound contact materials, there are other suitable products available. However, the lack of published data on their use within the pre-term population means that evidence-based practice cannot progress.

Wound assessment

This process to ensure that the most appropriate dressing is chosen (Miller, 1999) is as important in this group of patients as in any other.

A formal wound assessment chart should include the size and position of the injury and, although often subjective, the depth of the wound if possible. The colour of the wound bed — black, yellow, red or pink indicates the stage of healing, and recording the reduction in wound size can help to reassure the parents during this time. Malodour from the wound and the level of exudate can be subjective (small, medium, large). Photographic recordings of any injury and the stages of healing are helpful as injuries are often associated with litigation cases.

Risk assessment tools

It is important that the skin and wound care continues to develop in the area of neonatal nursing practice with specific tools developed to guide care provision.

Although there have been some skin assessment tools published, mainly from the USA, these have not been widely accepted due to the difference in practice.

The Braden scale has been adapted by adding the extra factors of tissue perfusion and oxygenation to make it more appropriate for children. It is known as the Braden Q score (Quigley and Curley, 1996); but, pre-term infants are not susceptible to typical pressure injuries so it is not a useful tool for this group.

Waterlow has adapted her Adult Risk Assessment for paediatric patients but, again, it was not felt to be appropriate for the very young (Waterlow, 1985, revised 1997).

The first specific neonatal skin risk assessment score was published by Huffines and Logsdon (1997). This is based on a small study of thirty-two neonates with a mean age of thirty-three weeks, and looked at six factors:

- general and physical condition
- mental state

- mobility, activity
- nutrition
- moisture.

Each factor has a score between 1–4, with 1 being the best and 4 the worst in each factor.

This system is useful in predicting the days most likely for skin breakdown, but does not give any direction on how to prevent this from happening or increasing in severity. This tool also grouped all the infants under twenty-eight weeks' gestation together but, in reality, there is a vast range in severity of illness, overall condition, and prognosis within this group of infants and, as such, this tool is not specific enough.

The most recent skin condition score was devised by Lund *et al* (2001), looking at three skin factors:

- dryness
- erythema
- breakdown/excoriation.

Each being scored 1–3 on a twice-weekly basis (1 being the best and 3 the worst).

This scoring system was introduced to monitor the improvements made following the introduction of evidence-based interventions across a large number of neonatal units. However, it is not specific enough to recommend a range of preventative measures which should be introduced at any given score to prevent the skin condition deteriorating further. This tool is not helpful for the very pre-term infant with their unique skin problems, but is useful as a more generalised tool for the more mature infant.

Without evidence-based nursing care practices which standardise care delivery, the development of a national risk assessment tool which will recommend specific interventions to prevent further deterioration is a long way off, and can only mean that optimal care is not yet being delivered.

References

Bravery K (1999) Paediatric intravenous therapy in practice. In: Dougherty L, Lamb J, eds. *Intravenous Therapy in Nursing Practice*. Churchill Livingstone, London

Connor JM, Soll RF, Edwards WH (2004) *Topical Ointment for Preventing Infection in Pre-term Infants*. Cochrane Database of Systematic Reviews:Art No CD001150

Gault D (1993) Extravasation injuries. *Br J Plastic Surg* **46**: 91–6

Harpin V, Rutter N (1983) Barrier properties of the newborn infants skin. *J Pediatr* **102**(3): 419–25

Harpin V, Rutter N (1985) Humidification of incubators. *Arch Dis Child* **60**: 210–24

Harpin V, Rutter N (1992) Percutaneous alcohol absorption and skin necrosis in a preterm infant. *Arch Dis Child* **57**: 477–9

Hecker J (1993) Survival of neonatal intravenous infusion sites. *Int J Pharmacy Practice* **12**: 82–5

Horii K, Lane A (2001) Evidence-based use of emollients in neonates. *Newborn Infant Nurs Rev* **1**(1): 21–4

Huffines B, Logsdon C (1997) The neonatal skin risk assessment scale for predicting skin breakdown in neonates. *Issues Comprehensive Pediatr Nurs* **20**: 103–14

Infection Control Nurses Association (2001) *Guidelines for Preventing Intravascular Catheter-related Infection*. ICNA, Fitwise Publication

Intravenous Nurses Society (2000) *Infiltration scale. Standards for infusion therapy*. Cambridge, MA. Cited in Royal College of Nursing (2003) Standards for Infusion Therapy. Royal College of Nursing: London

Irving V (2001) Reducing the risk of epidermal stripping in the neonatal population: an evaluation of an alcohol free barrier film. *J Neonatal Nurs* **7**(1): 5–8

Jackson A (1998) A battle in vein: infusion phlebitis. *Nurs Times* **94**(4): 68–71

Kuller J (1995) Skin care management of the low birth weight infant. In: Gunderson L, Kenner C, eds. *Care of the 24–25 Week Gestational Age Infant: A small baby protocol*. Nicu Inc CA

Linder N, Davidovitch N, Reichman B (1997) Topical iodine containing antiseptics and sub-clinical hypothyroidism in pre-term infants. *J Pediatr* **131**: 434–9

Lund C (1999) Prevention and management of infant skin breakdown. *Nurs Clin North Am* **34**(4): 907–20

Lund C, Oosborne J, Kuller J *et al* (2001) Neonatal skin care: clinical outcomes of the AWHONN/ NANN Evidence–based clinical practice guideline. *J Gynaecol Neonatal Nurs* **30**: 41–51

Malloy-McDonald M (1995) Skin Care for High Risk Neonates. *J Wound Ostomy Continence Nurs* **22**(4): 177–82

Miller M (1999) Wound assessment. In Miller M, Glover D, eds. *Wound Management: Theory and Practice*. Emap Healthcare Ltd, London

Nopper A, Kimberly A, Sookdeo-Drost S *et al* (1996) Topical ointment therapy benefits premature infants. *J Pediatr* **128**: 660–9

Pabst R, Starr K, Qaiyumi S *et al* (1999) The effect of application of Aquaphor on skin condition, fluid requirements, and bacterial colonization in very low birth weight infants. *J Perinatol* **19**(4): 278–83

Perez-woods R, Malloy MB (1992) Positioning and skin care of the low-birth-weight neonate. *NAACOG's Clinical Issues* **3**(1): 97–113

Quigley S, Curley M (1996) Skin integrity in the pediatric population: preventing and managing pressure ulcers. *J Soc Pediatr Nurses* **4**(1): 7–18

Rudy S (1991) From conception to birth: the development of skin and nursing care implications. *Dermatol Nurs* **3**(6): 381–90

Rutter N, Hull D (1979) Water Loss from the Skin of Term and Preterm Babies. *Arch Dis Child* **54**: 858–68

Rutter N, Hull D (1981) Effects of applying topical agents. *Arch Dis Child* **56**: 673–5

Rutter N (1996) The immature skin. *Eur J Pediatr* **155**: Supp 2S: 18–20

Schuren J, Becker A, Sibbgald RG (2005) A liquid film-forming acrylate for peri-wound protection: a systematic review and meta-analysis (3M™ Cavilon™ No Sting Barrier Film). *Int Wound J* **2**(3): 230–8

Smith R (1985) Prevention and Treatment of Extravasation. *Br J Parenteral Therapy* **6**: 114–18

Thomas S *et al* (1987) New approach to the management of extravasation injuries in neonates. *Pharmaceutical J* **239**: 584–5

Waterlow J (1997) Pressure sore risk assessment in children. *Paediatr Nurs* **9**(6): 21–4

Watkins A, Keogh E (1992) Alcohol burns in the neonate. *J Paediatr Child Health* **28**: 306–8

West D, Worobec S, Solomon L (1981) Pharmacology and Toxicology of Infant skin. *J Investigative Dermatol* **76**: 147–50

Winter G (1962) Formulation of the scab and the rate of epitheliasation in the skin of the domestic pig. *Nature* **193**: 293–4

Young T *et al* (1996) The use of a Hydrocolloid Dressing in the Treatment of Iatrogenic Neonatal Skin Trauma. In: Proceedings of the 6th European Conference on Advancement in Wound Management. Macmillan, London

INDEX